Broken Tees and Mended Hearts

A Life's Journey Serving
Wounded Warriors & Injured Spirits

By Judy Alvarez, PGA, LGPA

with Bob Denney

© 2011 by Judy Alvarez

Coleman
may the wind always be
at your Back!
JAlvarez

Contents

How To Use This Book

As an author and a golf professional, I'd love for you to read my book, cover to cover. In the interest of helping people to better help others, however, here's a quick tip on how you can best read and use this book. Either read sequentially or flip through the stories randomly if you like. Either way, I promise your time will be well spent. If you prefer, refer to the Index, which will direct you toward your specific needs.

While this is a book about golf and how the game can be used to motivate and inspire individuals with disabilities, it's more about the human spirit and how it overcomes and triumphs adversity and challenge. Whether you are a golf professional who wants to help others through your skills or someone who is looking for a way to help a friend return to the game of life, there's a story in here to inspire and guide you.

Warm-Ups

It's More than a Golf Lesson

Since World War II, The Professional Golfers Association of America has been a reservoir of service to those in the Armed Forces. From exhibition matches to aid the USO, to collecting dollars for a new fleet of ambulances, to supplying equipment, to developing programs for the returning veterans, PGA Professionals have been at the "front lines" on the range.

Today, PGA/LPGA Professionals like Judy Alvarez of Palm City, Florida, whose teaching career originated by learning from the golfers with disabilities, has risen to be one of the nation's finest in instructing our Wounded Warriors in how best to make a return to civilian life through golf.

In the years that I have known Judy, I have found her talents in communicating this game extend past the perimeter of a practice range. In the pages ahead, Judy invites us to observe both personal and emotional teaching experiences between a teacher and student. The golf instruction goes beyond take-home tips and branches into the mental and emotional stability for the student as well as his or her spouse or family.

From Judy's earliest memories as a golfer, we follow her through her own training and through the past decade as she developed her teaching skills that make a difficult game that much more understandable and enjoyable.

Perhaps you will find, as I did when helping Judy collect her vignettes, that there is so much more to each story. We are moved by the courage and life struggles of some remarkable human beings.

For the first time, an entire golf book is devoted to these proud men and women who have advanced — whether it is without a limb or with a multitude of physical injuries — and have reclaimed a large degree of normalcy in their lives.

Judy's career is a reflection of how powerful the game of golf is to healing broken spirits and opening a door to a new legion of consumers.

You will laugh, you will cry and you will discover, as did Judy, that the "physically challenged" are just like you and me.

As a golf professional once said, "Just call them by their name. That's all they ask."

Bob Denney

Palm Beach Gardens, Florida

A Message from Dennis Walters

"I just never assumed that I would not be able to play golf again, even though my doctors told me over and over that it was not even a remote possibility."

When Judy asked me to write this piece for her, I was very honored and only hoped that my words of wisdom and experience may give a better understanding of what it is like to be a physically challenged golfer. I actually think that I am in a much better position than most people to give this type of perspective. When I was a youngster, I learned to play golf in the traditional way, standing upright on my two legs and in most cases, I would always walk the 18 holes. I have always thought that one of the most enjoyable things about golf was that it gave you a chance to be outdoors in nature, listening to the birds, smelling the fresh cut lawn and getting exercise walking around the course.

I began my lifelong love affair with golf from the moment I first picked up a golf club at age six. I played golf as much as I could and always dreamed about joining the PGA TOUR after graduation from college. Unfortunately, that dream became a nightmare on July 21, 1974, when I was just 24 years old. I had a golf cart accident that left me paralyzed from the waist down.

While I was still in the hospital, I asked to have my golf clubs brought into the room so that I could hold them and keep working on my game while my body was healing. I just never assumed that I would not be able to play golf again, even though my doctors told me repeatedly that it was not even a remote possibility.

At the time of my accident, there was not a great deal of information available on golf for physically challenged individuals and everything I did to relearn the game was by trial and error, and believe me, there were plenty of errors and very trying times. I only wish that I had available to me back then all of the wonderful people like Judy to help me get back on my "feet."

My dad, Bucky, was one of the biggest influences in my life. He's the one who got me to take that first swing after my accident and although he had no formal training as a teacher, he was a casual golfer who tried to talk me through the relearning of my game. It's easy for a person to say that they understand what I was going through, but until they "walk in your shoes," there is just no way that they can fathom how difficult it is.

I still have been able to make golf my career of choice. I don't play on the PGA TOUR but I have my own tour now; THE DENNIS WALTERS GOLF SHOW has made more than 2,800 performances the last 34 years.

I travel all over the country encouraging others to reach for their dreams, strive for excellence, and try to do something that they did not think they could. My mission has always been to grow the game of golf for everyone, but especially those with disabilities.

Judy's path and mine crossed over 20 years ago because of our common interest — to make the game accessible to all. Judy's background as a golf instructor, her love of this great game, and her desire to make a difference have undoubtedly changed the lives of countless numbers of people. As with the teaching of anything, be it golf or education, patience, dedication, and understanding are key elements for the learning process.

I don't actually know what is more difficult for a teacher — having a physically challenged student who has never picked up a golf club, or someone like me, who was a standing golfer from a young age, who became disabled because of an accident. Judy has the ability for figuring out what is best for each individual she works with.

Judy's desire to make golf a game for everyone led to her being named by The PGA of America as the National Military Golf Trainer for The PGA Disabled Sports USA Military Golf Program. She is, as am I, involved with the Wounded Warrior Program.

Working with the unsung heroes, both men and women, who have returned from war with devastating injuries can be heart wrenching and difficult, but the rewards are far greater than one can imagine. Each day Judy gets the chance to change a life. When she sees a smile on someone's face the first time that they actually connect with that little white ball, it makes all the effort that she puts forth so worthwhile.

Golf can be a game for a lifetime and a big part of the rehabilitative process. In my case, golf was far better medicine than any pill I could take. There is so much more to the game of golf than just hitting the ball. Judy understands this and works tirelessly to help others understand that no matter what level they play the game, the result can be a life-changing experience. I know that everyone who reads this book or has the opportunity to meet and work with Judy will have a better understanding of the tremendous gift that she keeps on giving every day.

Dennis Walters, PGA Honorary Member
Jupiter, Florida

A Message from Major Dan Rooney, PGA Professional

As an F-16 pilot, I have served three tours of duty. I have witnessed great heroism and tragedy from the skies above Iraq. During those tours, I have been very blessed to cross paths with many exceptional patriots.

We have made great progress in the Middle East but not without great sacrifice. We have lost more than 5,000 troops and have more than 35,000 wounded veterans. These heroic warriors struggle every day to heal their physical and mental wounds, and golf has become an integral part of the healing process for many of our veterans.

When I think of golf's healing power, I am drawn back to a deployment in 2008 during which I was stationed at Joint Base Balad, Iraq. One of the great blessings of a deployment is the perspective it provides on the price of freedom.

We are all guilty of taking for granted the freedoms we enjoy every day. I fondly remember one evening when a small group of pilots discovered some beat-up clubs in a closet. We spent a couple hours having a highly competitive chipping contest. On that dusty evening it was more than golf, it was a connection to our lives back home. For a few moments we forgot we were in Iraq, and just enjoyed the game. Golf has the amazing power to transform us in the moment.

Though she has never donned a military uniform, Judy Alvarez loves and serves her country. A good friend, and great patriot, Judy is on a mission. Through golf she has brought fulfillment into the lives of thousands of golfers. But a handful of inspiring students are what distinguish her service to this nation.

Her dedication to disabled veterans is nothing short of inspirational. The game of golf is helping veterans reconnect with their family, friends, and their country.

Judy is providing the opportunity for our American heroes to heal their hearts and minds through golf. As a PGA/LPGA Teaching Professional, Judy has gone above and beyond the call of duty by serving disabled golfers.

Her distinguished career as a player and teacher are remarkable. Judy is truly a pioneer. From playing on the men's golf team in college, to serving on the board of directors for the Association of Disabled American Golfers, Judy has been blazing a trail in the world of golf for nearly three decades. Her vision, commitment, and passion are contagious. She is giving back to the game that has given each of us so much.

I am certain you will find *Broken Tees and Mended Hearts* resonates on many levels, elevating the knowledge of instructors about the chance to raise their own educational skills and serving as an inspiration to all who have never given a golf lesson but appreciate the quest to play the game. Judy's story is a glimpse of a career based on giving. A career dedicated to making the world a better place.

Judy and I share a common bond. We both realize that when you reach out to help someone in need, you are actually the one being helped.

Thank you, Judy, for your patriotism. I salute you for your service to this nation.

Maj. Dan Rooney, PGA

Broken Arrow, Oklahoma

Founder, Patriot Golf Day/Folds of Honor Foundation

My Incredible Journey Begins
by Judy Alvarez, PGA, LGPA Golf Professional

Every path starts somewhere. We all have a unique beginning to our professional journeys; mine began some 20 years ago. The vignettes that follow will take you down a variety of fairways as you "share the golf cart" with me as a golf instructor. The journey has afforded me countless rewarding relationships with many wonderful people.

After a few years working as an assistant golf professional in the early 1990s, I received a telephone call from two of these special people, PGA Professional Marybeth Corrigan and Tom Haase, offering me the opportunity to take over the head golf professional position at a facility in Palm Beach County, Florida. In addition to my many responsibilities of managing an 18-hole public golf course, I would also be overseeing a staff of 28, owning a retail golf store and an aqua driving range, conducting weekly tournaments and leagues, and giving daily lessons.

During my professional career, few days ever pass when I am not asked, "How did you get started teaching golf to the disabled or injured?" and, "How do you teach them?"

The truth is that while working at this public course, I had to step up to the starting line. One component of my instructional program was teaching a weekly adaptive golf class.

Although my new position would begin on a Monday and I was excited and overwhelmed with everything I had to do, this adaptive golf class that I had to teach at the end of the week was weighing in the back of my mind. I had experience teaching, but not to a group of people with disabilities. Naturally, I was a bit apprehensive.

Aware that my current education as a golf instructor did not fully prepare me for teaching an extraordinary group of golfers, I set out on a research mission and arrived in Colorado to witness the work of the Association of Disabled American Golfers. They were hosting their annual golf tournament, pairing golfers with and without disabilities.

This truly was the spark that ignited my teaching career. I had never seen so many enthusiastic golfers with injuries, using an assortment of assistive devices and adaptive equipment, all in one place.

I returned to South Florida armed with an arsenal of modified swing techniques and an expanded library of teaching aid resources, including something called a "single-rider" golf cart. Participating in this event inspired me to start my own able-bodied/disabled-bodied golf event.

Concurrently, during the 1990s, the Americans with Disabilities Act was passed to eliminate discrimination against people with disabilities. This created a great deal of activity in our country, the golf industry, and, most importantly to me, in the accessible world of golf.

My experiences with this eager golfing population inspired me to tell their story, which I hope will now inspire you. These vignettes are about mothers and fathers, sons and daughters, sisters and brothers, your neighbors and co-workers, survivors, veterans of war and members of local communities whose careers were disrupted, some to protect our country's freedom.

These stories exemplify living each day to the fullest in spite of an injury, defying death, overcoming emotional setbacks and illness, and personal and family triumphs. They show us just how much the human body and soul can endure through physical, mental and emotional trauma and still find the will to live.

You will learn how a cast of family and friends, strangers and neighbors, therapists, nurses and doctors, and golf instructors came to support those in need, helping them overcome adversity.

I hope this book will encourage you as much as the subject matter has helped me. Through my experiences, I began to understand that the game of golf could be a therapeutic and rehabilitative tool, a healer, and a means to improve one's quality of life. Yes, it's true, golf can help save lives.

I feel that these stories will provide inspiration and motivation to those who are living with disabilities or know someone with an injury. My hope is that others will be inspired when they learn of the extraordinary circumstances my students have had to negotiate with minimal complaint. Perhaps your heart may feel an extra beat as you meet the courageous people who populate these stories and inspire me daily. Some things in life are priceless and one can never put a price tag on the companionship, friendship, sharing and personal growth found in these anecdotes.

Judy Alvarez, PGA/LPGA Golf Professional

The Front Nine

Brighter Fairways

It was about 3:30 p.m. on a sun-splashed Saturday when I opened up the book on my first accessible golf class. It was as if someone had rolled out a red carpet. Around the corner of the clubhouse my group started arriving, one by one. There was Rob, who had suffered a stroke, limping with the assistance of a quad cane. He was followed by Eugene, whose cerebral palsy caused him to shuffle his legs from side to side with very little range of motion. Dave, Gail, and Jared soon rolled up in both manual and electric wheelchairs.

Kristen, one of the smallest people I had ever met, arrived with a megawatt smile. Then there was Fritz, a happy-go-lucky young man wearing thick-rimmed glasses who ran with an odd gait straight past us as if we did not exist, making a beeline for the practice range. He was on a mission to hit balls. In a very short time, his enthusiasm became infectious.

I kept my nerves and fears tucked underneath my visor as I stepped into the realm of the unknown. I think most golf instructors would agree that unless you have had experience teaching golfers with disabilities, you are going to feel like a nervous student pilot in their company.

I kept thinking, out of innocence and ignorance, "What happens if I say the wrong thing, if I insult or offend someone?" In just a short time, my uneasiness was over.

After introductions, everyone worked their way up to the semi-circular aqua practice range and began hitting balls. Moving from station to station, I noticed something different from my "conventional" classes. The pace was slower. There were extra people, family members and friends, to assist each student.

I observed heaps of chairs, a supply of umbrellas, many extra buckets of balls, an odd-looking golf cart with a bench seat removed and replaced by a swivel seat, hitting mats, shorter clubs, clubs with flexible shafts, grabbers and more.

I also realized that I had to change hats and thought processes for each person I coached. In one station, the student was swinging from a seated position. The student in the next station was swinging with only one arm, and in another station, there was a fellow swinging with braces on both of his legs. It was the most unconventional experience I had ever encountered as a golf instructor.

I took a few deep breaths and thought, "I can do this! I should be able to figure out a way to help each of them to hit balls successfully." After all, if they were going to take time out of their schedules and commit to this class every week, the least I could do was be open-minded and figure out a way to help them.

It was at this point in my teaching career that I realized it was not my side of the ball that was important; it was theirs!

Outgoing and fun-loving Dave, a Long Island native, had become a paraplegic after being hit by a car while riding his bike home from a Little League baseball game when he was only 10 years old. As an adult, he enjoyed many sports, including tennis, but really loved attending golf classes and hanging out with everyone. He said, "I feel like this class is a huge stress reliever and we're always laughing." Looking away, he added, "The only drawback is that since I am strapped in to the golf cart on this swivel seat, my legs just dangle and I need someone to tee up the ball for me. I like being independent. So I either need help or I use the grabber and tee up the ball myself."

There was lanky Rob, who always wore his baseball cap and was escorted by his wife and two children for encouragement. A stroke on the left side forced Rob to swing with only his right arm. Since stamina was an issue, he needed many visits to the bench as a reprieve between shots. I remember Rob saying, "Well, it's not going far, but at least it's going straight." The dream, wish and goal of all golfers!

Eugene, a black-haired lefty in his mid-twenties, had cerebral palsy. He was so excited when he hit the ball, cresting it into the air maybe 60 yards. He got the biggest kick out of watching the ball splash into the water! Granted, this distance would not be acceptable for the majority of golfers out there, but not everyone was walking in Eugene's shoes. "I blistered the ball, Coach Judy," he would proudly declare.

Kristen, just 42 inches tall due to spina bifida and in her late 20s, clocked the ball all of 20 yards. She told me, "Judy, when we go onto the golf course, I aim for the cart path because I get more distance. I need what I can get."

Gail, a graduate of the University of Delaware who taught physical education, had a spinal cord disease and never complained about where the ball went. She was content just swinging away and enjoying her time, and would let out a contagious laugh. "Judy, want to hear a joke?" was her favorite line. Gail lived a short but full life, passing away early due to health complications.

Our slim Jared, with the aid of his loving mom, dad and younger brother, hit balls from his electric wheelchair. His neurological disorder curbed his speech, but not his enthusiasm. I will never forget the incredible bonding among that family.

Never have I witnessed a person so addicted to the game of golf as Fritz. Anyone who knew him would agree with me. A stout, robust young man in his late teens, he was always accompanied by his mom and older brother. Although he had a neurological disorder and was to some degree mentally challenged, Fritz was one of the most bubbly, energetic young men I'd ever met. It was clear by his entrance to class that this session was the highlight of his week. Like an addict, he could never get enough of hitting golf balls. An awkward swing at best, his hand-eye coordination took over and propelled the ball with surprising accuracy. Fritz had a short attention span and would always say, "Look, Coach Judy! Watch what I can do." It was as if his life depended on the shot.

I was so pumped up after this class! I felt a connection to these people and a renewed bond with the game of golf, which I now viewed from a whole new perspective. These students showed me that the game was much more than just hitting the golf ball far or shooting the lowest score. It was about having fun and laughing, overcoming barriers, sharing and spending quality time with one other.

I looked back and wondered why I had been so worried. My new students thanked me for having a good time and then told me I had done a great job teaching their class. It was as if they were coaching me and I had passed the test. I wondered who was teaching whom? We all felt better about ourselves following our Saturday session.

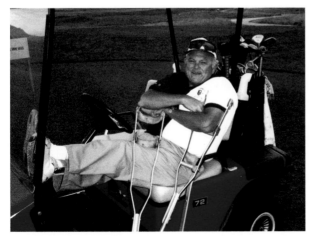

Greg Jones. (Picture courtesy of Vicki Chase)

Inspired by this wonderful group of golfers, I was determined to learn more about opportunities for this special population.

My search brought me to Denver in the early 1990s, where I met Greg Jones. This cheery and stocky Executive Director for the Association of Disabled American Golfers invited me to play in their annual two-day tournament, pairing golfers with and without disabilities. Since I was new to teaching accessible golf programs, this event caught my interest.

Have you ever played golf with someone with a disability or competed in a golf tournament where half the field has an injury and they are out to take your money? Those same golf partners of yours may be disabled, but they are there to play some golf. You know, chase the ball for a few hours, win a few side bets, see if they're lucky enough for closest to the pin or longest drive and throw down a few with their buddies at the 19th hole.

A beautiful Rocky Mountain sunrise formed a stunning backdrop for the practice range on opening day. I had never experienced an event of this magnitude. The range was filled to capacity with golfers with odd-looking stances, lined up and hitting balls. Maybe I shouldn't say "odd," but they were certainly set-ups and swing motions I had never seen before. They were just doing whatever it took to hit the ball. As I looked around, I saw the staging area filled with strange but well-designed looking golf carts with only one seat; and adjacent to them were trailers and wheelchairs.

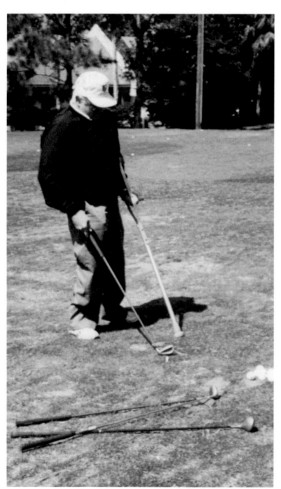

Greg Jones getting ready to swing.

Tom Houston, paralyzed from the waist down, was hitting balls from a stand-up position with the use of a motorized "HiRider," a specially adapted golf cart that he designed himself. He had a fabulous backswing and follow through. Greg, who had post-polio syndrome, was supporting himself on one crutch while swinging with one arm. Golfers on one leg were hitting balls with uncanny balance. Others were swinging away with one arm, hitting the ball farther than I could ever have done with two arms. I saw a double amputee hitting balls from a wheelchair. There were homemade and store-bought devices attaching golfers to their clubs and something new to the golf industry — those single rider golf carts.

I followed the advice which I always give to my own students and became a sponge, soaking up the many unconventional but successful methods of hitting golf balls. I had never been in an amphitheater quite like this, and realized the unlimited possibilities for the injured to enjoy the game of golf.

I wondered how these golfers were going to tackle the foothills and steep slopes on the outskirts of Denver. After the shock wore off, I realized there was some serious competition surrounding me and that hills and wheelchairs did not matter; golf mattered. As PGA Professional Pam Elders and long-time friend said while playing in this same event, "If you want something bad enough, you will figure out a way to do it. And that's exactly what I observed."

I watched as golfers tackled bunkers with a single-rider golf cart; I watched as a player drove from shot to shot by maneuvering his HiRider up a trailer hitched to the back of a golf cart. I observed a golfer in a wheelchair hold onto the side of a golf cart to get to his next lie. I not only witnessed a single-rider golf cart parked on the fringe of the green so someone could chip on, this unique cart also drove across a putting green. My circuits were on overload.

And then my brain processed it all. I realized that the game of golf is inclusionary, an equalizer, and has the potential to bring everyone together regardless of ability. Some of these golfers may have lost their legs or were paralyzed, but they were there to win and everyone was having a good time. We were all there for the same reasons: to have fun outdoors, escape the worries of the world, share in the fellowship and appreciation of friends, and, of course, for some healthy competition!

This experience inspired me to start my own tournament, the Brighter Fairways Classic, which ran successfully and enthusiastically for six years, pairing golfers with and without disabilities. Running such a large event required a lot of help, so I recruited my able-bodied golf students, to whom I owe a great "thank you." It was special to me to witness able-bodied golfers grow, both as people and as golfers. I have watched many non-injured golfers practice without a purpose and comment that they cannot do this or that. What they learned by volunteering was that their lives were not that bad after all. They found a greater appreciation for their own games.

It has occurred to me that although I am not a medical doctor and cannot write prescriptions for medication, as a golf instructor I can prescribe a game that can foster growth and enhance someone's life. That is a PGA/LPGA teaching professional's prescription; a home remedy, if you will.

As I reflected on this accessible golf experience, I became acutely aware of many things. Primarily, I needed to focus more on a person's abilities than disabilities. I realized that it doesn't matter if someone is swinging on one or two legs, with one or two arms, sitting or standing, using a regular-length club or one 24 inches, the game of golf is a wonderful equalizer.

I have learned that providing a foundation to help someone learn about him or herself and build their self-confidence is very important. It has become apparent to me that the environment for social interaction, for loved ones spending quality time together and sharing in the camaraderie of sport, especially after a life-changing injury, is equally important.

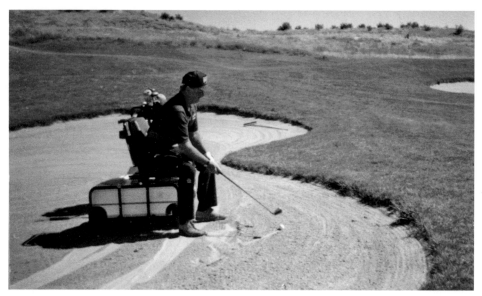

Dave White lining up his bunker shot.

Friendship and Freedom on the Links
"Golf gave me back my sense of dignity and self-worth."

Over the years, many students have rolled into my office seeking golf lessons. Each arrives bearing different attitudes and expectations and progressing through different phases of recovery: physically, mentally or emotionally. As a golf instructor who specializes in working with disabled golfers, I have always looked forward to these special sessions.

I first met Herb and his wife, Sue, at a local club in Port St. Lucie, Florida, approximately two years after his accident. Herb is a wonderful man with a contagious laugh and a great sense of humor. A successful ophthalmologist with a deep love for the game of golf, his life turned upside down one day when a staph infection left him paralyzed after a successful coronary bypass surgery.

As with all permanent injuries, this loving couple, like so many others, faced an altered lifestyle, including a home and office that had to be made disabled-friendly. They purchased a handicap conversion van to accommodate Herb's wheelchair. Everyday tasks had to be re-learned while Herb's psyche was dealing with the stages of denial, anger, bargaining, depression and acceptance of his paralysis.

Although it is different for every individual who has sustained a life-changing injury, at some point Herb and Sue were determined to pick up the pieces of their lives and resume their recreational activities. In Herb's case it was golf, but he was unsure how to return since he had only played from a traditional standing position.

His long time dear friends told him that I taught golfers with disabilities and suggested that he give me a call. I didn't realize then the impact this one telephone call would have on all of us — a call that turned into a lifetime friendship. It didn't occur to me that an ordinary sport — golf — would have such an extraordinary outcome.

Having worked with many injured golfers, I knew Herb would be a great candidate as long as he brought with him two main ingredients — an open mind and the right attitude. Since he had overcome redoing his life after his paralysis, I hoped hitting golf balls would seem benign. The question was, would it meet his expectations? As a golf teacher, I cannot control that. I can only provide a safe, fun learning environment to springboard students to new experiences and self-discovery.

Upon their arrival for our first lesson, I watched the couple's chemistry and teamwork as they entered the parking lot area and rolled into my office.

Their teamwork would be critical in creating a solid foundation for starting off on the right foot in building a new chapter in their lives together. If there was any apprehension — fear of failing, falling down, or people staring at him — Herb's enthusiastic attitude overshadowed all of it. After sitting down and sharing with each other for a while, it became clear that Herb's open-mindedness, determination, and desire were on board and accounted for.

Sue was as deeply interested and attentive, believing that if she could get her husband involved with golf again, it would elevate his spirits and they could both go back to playing golf — something they had really enjoyed doing together.

Sue's commitment illustrates something that's too often forgotten in these scenarios — the loved ones of the injured. Their lives are changed also. Sue inherited the role of caregiver like so many others who serve injured loved ones. For health reasons and camaraderie, it was important that Sue see Herb become connected with the game of golf once again.

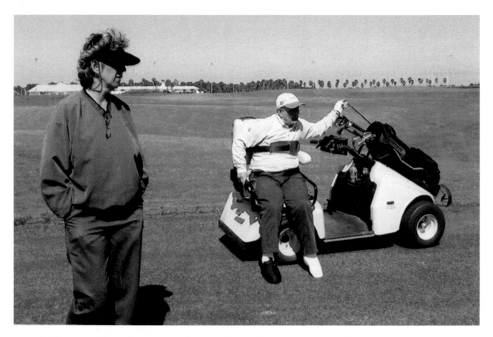

Coach Alvarez and Herb sizing up the next shot. (Picture courtesy of Herb Heins)

From experience, I knew that there are a variety of ways to teach a golf swing to someone in a seated position. It just takes some experimenting based upon the student's previous skill level, expectations and attitude.

I showed Herb multiple ways to hit balls from a seated position. First, we experimented with his wheelchair facing the ball with a traditional set-up position, using a somewhat flatter club. We tried swinging with one arm from the side of his chair using a three-wood about 24 inches long. Then I showed Herb the method that won him over — hitting balls while strapped into a single-rider golf cart. The cart had an electronic swivel seat capable of moving him up and down and from side to side, which afforded the greatest range of motion.

Herb's reaction was first-class; even better was his wife's surprise when she saw him strike the ball. This was definitely the "moment of truth" that we hopefully all encounter when we realize there is something that can help us to overcome some of life's tragedies.

A single-rider golf cart designed to help people with paralysis was Herb's link to freedom. The game of golf rejuvenated Herb and Sue and added another dimension to their social lives. They had sorely missed being outdoors in the fresh air, getting some exercise and spending time together.

Had it not been for this cart, Herb would not have had the independence and freedom to hit balls on the range, putt on the green or chase the ball on the golf course. More importantly,

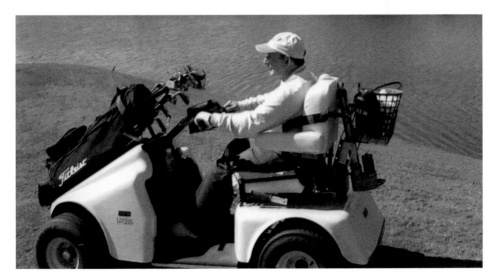

Herb in his single-rider golf cart, one tool that enabled him to get back into the game. (Picture courtesy of Herb Heins)

being able to get around on his own had restored his sense of self-worth and dignity.

His excitement and exhilaration were overwhelming. His eyes sparkled with enthusiasm. Somewhat apprehensive in the beginning, he knew that being a part of society again was better than any hole–in-one. Since this experience, Herb and Sue are playing golf together again. Herb has purchased his own single-rider cart and a set of custom made flatter golf clubs. Even Sue's game, which went on hiatus after Herb's injury, has gotten back on track.

From the clubhouse one day I observed Herb playing golf in his single-rider cart, sharing time with Sue. This was another reminder of how the game can have such a remarkable impact on people's lives. Golf was the link to my wonderful friendship with Herb and Sue, and their link to renewed freedom and fun. I am honored to know them.

That image of Herb will be forever seared into my mind — him rolling away in his special golf cart, a reborn golfer with a new attitude and a happy, loving wife strolling beside him, forever grateful for that phone call that helped him to heal.

Life in a Rear View Mirror
"You'll probably be confined to a wheelchair within five years.
You'll never walk again."

As the shocking words came out of her doctor's mouth, it was as if Vicki went deaf. She could see her doctor talking to her but couldn't hear a word he was saying. The only thing Vicki heard were echoes pounding in her head. He told her, "You have reflex sympathetic dystrophy, which is an injury to your right leg that will diminish your lower body stability and balance. We are going to have to insert a computerized Internal Peripheral Nerve stimulator wired to your right hip so it can send electrodes behind your knee to shock the nerve endings to reduce pain. Plan on being in a wheelchair within five years."

How could this be happening? This just was not acceptable. The day of her accident was like any other day on the job for Vicki. One minute she had been conducting business as usual, the next, some heavy boxes fell on her foot and she was being rushed to the hospital. Hearing this life-altering news from her doctor was like a bad dream! How could her life have changed in the blink of an eye? She thought her life would never be the same.

What would her future hold? Confined to a wheelchair? She was a grown woman in her mid-thirties who was now going to have to learn to walk all over again?

At this point in her life, she thought she would be doing other things, not learning how to put one foot in front of the other, learning how to get in and out of bed again, or how to rise from a sitting position. She was supposed to be traveling the world, enjoying family, friends and days on the beach. How could life be so fragile?

After numerous surgeries, Vicki underwent months of follow-up rehab. "For what?" she asked herself. She still had shortness of breath, felt weak and limped along with the aid of a cane. She wondered if this was how the rest of her life was going to be.

A concerned friend saw Vicki's fire and passion for life fading away, stifled by depression and medication and clouded by sadness. An avid golfer, this friend suggested that Vicki try playing golf to get outdoors in the fresh air. Vicki replied, "I don't play golf. What good would that do? And besides, that's not something I can do in my condition anyway."

Almost to the day of the fifth anniversary of hearing that she would be in a wheelchair for the rest of her life, Vicki climbed out of the golf cart and, with cane in hand, limped up the low-graded hill to a picturesque practice range for her first golf lesson.

Something wondrous transpired that day on the driving range in Margate, Florida. Vicki says, "I am a firm believer that people walk in and out of our lives for a greater purpose." In Vicki's case, that moment was meeting her new golf instructor.

We sat on a wooden bench beneath a huge willow tree, exchanged information and enlightened each other about our backgrounds. Then we designed a plan that included short- and long-term goals.

Over the next few weeks, we began exploring different swing motions. Since Vicki, who plays right-handed, was unable do the typical cookie-cutter swing, a flat-footed swing provided the best outcome — both for trusting that she wouldn't fall down and for maximizing the flight of the ball. Vicki's swing evolved, allowing her lower body to stay still while her upper body turned on a more stable foundation. Here we found another golf swing to adapt to a unique disability. Vicki was on her way to advancing the ball to the point where she would be able to play the game with joy and dignity.

Vicki began to realize that golf was a treatment that no amount of medication could provide. As volcanic courage and perseverance slowly erupted from within her, things started to change. It was a little overwhelming and I do not think she really had a grasp on it at the time, but something was happening.

Her balance started stabilizing. Her endurance increased. She did not tire as quickly, and, best of all, her enthusiasm to do more outdoor activities increased. She started to feel more confidence in herself. She began to socialize more — something she really had not had the desire to do since her injury.

Golf became a healing vehicle for Vicki, proving her doctors wrong. "I was not destined to be a cripple," she states. She knew she had limitations but was not going to let them stop her. She would continue to walk, even with pain and discomfort.

Taking her initial steps from the practice range to the first tee was very much like the leader walking up the dogleg-right 18th hole at Augusta National. With nerves of steel, Vicki hunkered down and took a flat-footed swing, propelling that white ball down the middle of the fern-colored fairway. She was beaming with excitement. She took pride in ownership of the work she had put into her game just to pull off this one shot.

A few weeks later, I was thrilled when Vicki accepted my invitation to join me as my playing partner in the annual able-bodied/disabled-bodied two-day golf tournament, hosted at the time by the Association of Disabled American Golfers in Denver, Colorado.

I knew if she participated in this event, not only would it help her self-esteem, she would also see that there is a fulfilling world out there waiting for her, even with an injury.

Over the next six months, we had a great deal of work to do to get Vicki's game in shape. Vicki understood that with daily progress also came obstacles and temporary setbacks. She did not give up and continued to drive forward, seeing how far she could push herself without falling over and still hit the ball successfully. What staying power!

Once we arrived to the mountainous golf course located roughly 25 miles west of Denver, Vicki was captivated by her eye-opening experience. She revealed, "I witnessed so many golfers in situations far worse than mine. I saw golfers swinging out of machines to help them stand or sit up and, also, many with less mobility than I who could actually do more." She started purging herself of the "poor pitiful me" syndrome.

Vicki's exposure to this sold-out event 2,500 miles west of her Florida home made her realize that life had much to offer her in spite of her permanent injury. For the first time in years, her dreary yesterdays of indifference and depressing gray turned to colorful tomorrows of vitality and vibrancy. She realized, "If they could do it, so can I."

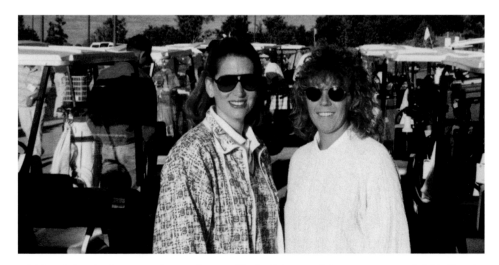

Vicki and Coach Alvarez getting ready to tackle the fairways. (Picture courtesy of Vicki Chase)

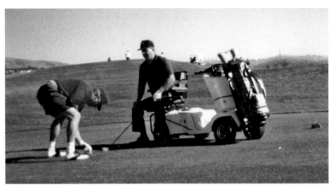

Larry Allen helping his teammate Dave White tee up the ball.

As it turned out, walking with the assistance of her cane to the ball on the golf course became secondary to the side bet our team had with two new friends/competitors, Larry and Dave, who played in our group the first day. Our focus was on beating the boys. After a few hours of chasing the ball we all met at the "19th" hole to compare scores. We won! It was like winning our own Masters!

To this day, Vicki still holds a special place in her heart for the game of golf. A game she had never before played before her life-altering injury. With conviction in her voice, Vicki states, "For those who fail to comprehend why people play golf, you must try it for yourself. You really don't know what you are missing. Trust me, there will be no more looking at your life in a rear-view mirror. You won't look back, you won't regret it, and you'll wish you picked it up years ago."

In addition to making new friends on the fairways, Vicki renewed her passion for photography, taking many beautiful pictures of scenery around the world.

Vicki and I returned to Colorado for the next three years to play as partners. Although we did not capture our division title, what we won was substantially greater than any trophy. "Golf has changed my life completely," said Vicki, "and you never know where it'll take you."

A Stroke of Good Fortune
"Thank you, golf. You saved my life."

She teed up the ball, drew the club back, and smacked it down the left side of the fairway. It didn't go as far as it used to, but it was still in the short grass closer to the hole. Not bad considering that she did it with only one arm. She smiled and felt so much better knowing she was back on a golf course. For quite some time, Shirley, a strong and fit woman in her early fifties, who had the good fortune to retire young, questioned if she would ever get back to the fairways.

Shirley was an avid golfer who loved the game. She teed up whenever and wherever she could. She would play in the women's league, member-guest events, local outings and in the late afternoon just before sunset. She had taken lessons from me throughout the years and always aspired to be better at hitting the ball and lowering her score. Shirley was one of those rare individuals who had a true appreciation and respect for the sport.

One morning just prior to Thanksgiving, Shirley's life was forever changed in a blink of an eye. She went from sipping coffee and checking e-mails to being rushed to the hospital by ambulance.

Her family gathered around as the doctors went to work. The diagnosis of an ischemic stroke on her left side made her passion for life — and golf — as distant as Pebble Beach is from St. Andrews. Crying, shaking, her mouth twisted as a tumble of words slurred. Her family braced for the worst.

While golf became a fading memory, frustration and anger became her constant companions. She wondered how this could have happened to her. One minute she was in good health and the next minute she was learning how to walk and talk again. Much later, Shirley would remark, "Defeat was not in my vocabulary and I had to persevere." After all, this was just a set-back. She was not a quitter and as hard as things seemed, she had always drawn upon her infinite reserve of will to overcome so much adversity. Perhaps this is why Shirley had always experienced success as a golfer.

What she wouldn't give to be practicing her putting. Instead she was relearning how to place one foot in front of the other, walking up and down a flight of stairs and supporting herself on bars. What she wouldn't give to be out in the fresh air instead of being cooped up inside, rehabilitating. It was all she could do as she regained her strength to just stand and walk again. She went from chasing golf balls to dodging therapists as they perused her through the halls of the rehab center.

Slowly, as each day of physical, occupational and speech therapy unfolded, she found herself closer to making the turn to a green that lay just ahead. She said, "I don't care if I walk perfectly, I just want to go back to playing golf again."

Shirley saw the value of golf in her rehabilitation and wanted to figure out how to play golf swinging with just one arm. With today's medical insurance battles, therapy sessions are becoming limited, causing patients to pay out-of-pocket expenses much sooner than anticipated. It seemed incredibly logical to become involved in a golf program as early as possible in order to expedite her therapy. Once she had clearance from her doctor, Shirley and I sat down and mapped out a plan.

The game of golf is a wonderful therapeutic tool for a "stroker" to get back into the swing of things, both on and off the golf course. Granted, rehab wasn't going to "cure" her stroke; however, it did teach Shirley how to manage herself for the best long-term outcome. Similar to everyone who has suffered a stroke, Shirley was given these simple, yet difficult, marching orders for the remainder of her life: "Therapy will end at some point. You're going to have to have the discipline to continue your exercises."

As a "stroker," what better place to continue a "health maintenance" program than outside in the fresh air on a golf course? Just about every aspect of the game challenged Shirley, similar to everything she had been working on while in rehab. From sitting, standing and walking, to working on balance and transferring her weight, Shirley was challenged. Concentration, patience, building endurance, developing her hand-eye coordination and fine motor skills (finger, hands and arms), are all necessary for playing on a golf course, and beneficial as rehabilitation exercises.

For months, with the help of loved ones, she worked on her golf exercises, which would help her know how to play again using only one side of her body. She started small, with putting and getting in and out of a golf cart. The seemingly simple task of walking to and from the ball proved to be very taxing and frustrating. In time, her stamina improved. Shirley graduated to hitting balls off tees on the driving range and eventually worked her way onto the golf course.

There were many days when Shirley's practice sessions resembled a ping pong match: quitting versus perseverance. She even questioned what she was doing and evaluated its value. Her will to succeed out-weighed giving up. Perseverance won out.

Her inner strength was inspirational as she transferred her positive attitude to other people who have had a stroke or simply think golf is too difficult a sport to play. She wasn't about to let her stroke affect her ability to play golf, albeit in a style which was all her own.

The human body is an amazing machine, one which can be retrained and rehabilitated. Over time Shirley learned the critical life skills necessary to return to her everyday ways. An encouraged Shirley says, "I hope you find and create a partnership with a local golf professional who will teach you a modified swing and game like I did."

For all those people that have had a stroke or those who have suffered a similar plight, the golf course invites you with open arms. If Shirley did it, so can you. The game of golf is within reach of anyone

As the blossoms of spring appeared along with her new swing, Shirley poked another one down the fairway; you could hear her mutter as she got herself into the cart and rode away with her daughter, "Thank you, golf; you've saved my life!"

What Golf Teaches Us About A Guy Named Stan

"Golf doesn't discriminate against cancer."

From its roots, the sport of golf is not designed to judge if you hit the ball from tee to green in a single shot on a par-4 or just dribble it out some 50 yards. It is unimportant what side of the ball you're swinging from. It does not matter if you are a hacker or a tour professional, young or old, male or female, lefty or righty, or whether you are playing in Utah or Europe. The game is simply non-judgmental.

It doesn't matter if you are utilizing clubs that are the latest and greatest pieces of technology or hand-me-downs. It doesn't discriminate if you are swinging on one leg or two, or from a seated or standing position. Best of all, golf was not created to judge your skill level. What golf does provide are the most simple, yet most meaningful opportunities for all participants.

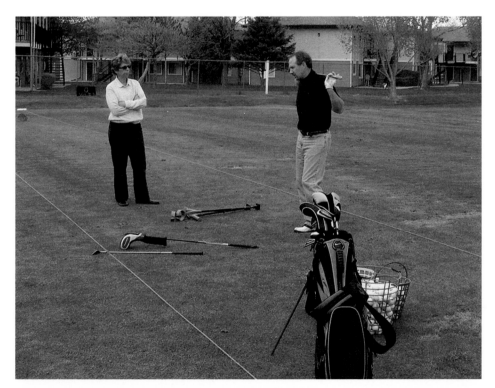

Stan and Judy discussing his golf swing.

Poised in the basin of the Salt Lake Valley surrounded by white-capped mountain peaks, I saw my playing field from a fresh perspective. It was a cool spring day when I met Stan at the oasis. Stan was the man who showed me that golf has no regard if his hip and femur bone were taken away by bone cancer, leaving no bones connecting his left leg to his left hip and no bone connecting his pelvis to his knee.

Stan is still strolling, or I should say now rolling, down the tree-lined fairways and has actually lowered his handicap (golf handicap, that is) since he has devoted more time to his short game. For some of us, once a round of golf is over, we head home to mow the lawn or do household chores — not Stan. He goes home to bed and pretty much stays there and recuperates for the rest of the day.

Playing a round of golf wears him out. If you ask Stan if it's worth it, he would reply, "You bet it is. Just because I can't change or cure the medical issues life has dealt me doesn't mean I should stop playing." What golf has done is provide him with a renewed opportunity to experience the joy and benefits that come from playing the game. His dangling left leg may

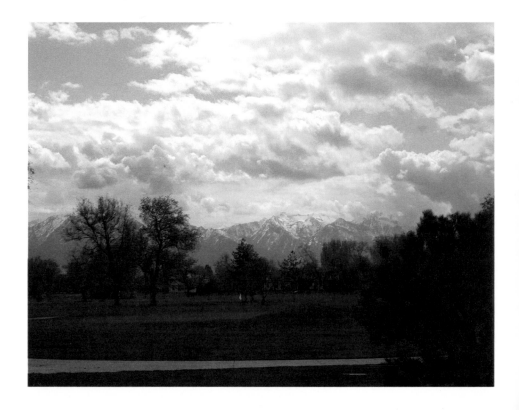

be non-weight-bearing and cause him to have an unorthodox swing; however, none of this diminishes his enthusiasm and sense of fulfillment out on the course.

The sensational feat about playing golf is that the ball doesn't know if Stan has the perfect swing, or if he is battling bone cancer and is missing the majority of his hip. As long as Stan gets the clubface back to the ball rather squarely at a fast pace, the ball is going forward toward the target.

Sure, he needs to use a crutch as his "third leg" to move around and get into his set-up position, but there are all sorts of people tackling this sport who have peculiar-looking swings. I witnessed Stan's shots soar high and far, and once it left his club face it looked just like all the other golf shots.

Playing with his family is now one of the highlights of Stan's day. In fact, for years Stan tried to get his son and daughter to play golf with him, but they were always involved in other sports or didn't have time. Cancer changed family priorities. Now Stan gets to tee it up with his son and daughter, outings he really enjoys.

After spending time with Stan, I thought of him as a regular guy, not someone with a disability. Every person deserves a chance to play golf, Stan was no exception. In the purest form, he should be able to play just like the "best" of them.

They Don't Give Us One-Armed Tee Boxes

"Golf is a great getaway, especially on those 'one-armed' days."

Four days prior to beginning his freshman year of college, and intent on trying out as a walk-on for the 1994 college baseball season, tragedy struck Jeff. An industrial accident took the right arm of this shortstop and second baseman, from above the elbow, ending his hopes and dreams of playing baseball.

Anyone who has suffered a serious accident knows well how the medical bills pile up. The local community gathered to support Jeff and his family by hosting a golf tournament to raise funds to offset those medical expenses.

Late in the round, one of the tournament participants, leaning over a lengthy putt, said to Jeff, "Why don't you putt this out for me? I don't feel like doing it." So, Jeff traded the seven-foot flagstick he was holding for a two-ball putter. Jeff's dad, standing nearby, noticed a look in his son's eyes he had not seen since Jeff lost his arm. The sparkle had returned — a look of desire; that "competitive glaze."

For months, father and son worked on Jeff's short game. When he had built sufficient strength, Jeff started to swing a driver with his left arm from a right-handed swing position. Jeff played his first round of golf one year to the day after his accident!

That day, Jeff went from holding a flagstick for others to getting himself back into the game of golf. Today, on average, Jeff shoots in the high 70s to low 80s. In the fall of 2009, he tested his competitive edge and teed it up for the first time in the North American One Armed National Championship held in Palm Beach, Florida.

Over the years many have asked Jeff how the game of golf helped him. His reply is always simple and from the heart: "It gave me that competitive outlet that was taken away from me when I lost my ability to play baseball." With his dreams shattered, he thought his life was over. The mental pain was a silent killer, leaving him depressed and suicidal. One putt helped turn his life around.

Jeff had always known that playing baseball would eventually end after college and wondered what he would do. It never occurred to him that he would be playing golf, let alone with one arm, or as he calls it, "backhanded" "Golf is a sport you can play until you just can't do it anymore. Age and injury are irrelevant; it's a sport you can do forever," he said.

It's a great get-away, too, on those "one-armed" days, as Jeff calls them, when he needs to lift his spirits, those days that he becomes frustrated because he can't do the things he would like to because they require two arms. On those days he heads out to the driving range and swings his driver to see just how far he can hit that ball.

Although it is much more difficult to swing with one arm, it can be done, and Jeff has found it a lot of fun. So much fun, that he set a world record in 2006 for the longest carry of a golf ball in the air — 258 yards, 2 feet, 4 inches! Not bad for a right-hander who swings backhanded across his body. If you witnessed his swing, you would marvel at its textbook-quality.

Jeff has totally embraced the game and now coaches golf at a Bible college in Oklahoma. He shares with his players how strength, courage and confidence got him through his initial ordeal and continues to help him through tough times. He is an inspiration to his players and a powerful advocate for the game he loves.

No, golf courses don't come packaged with tee boxes designed for one-armed golfers. But, Jeff will challenge anyone to a game of golf and show just how priceless the game has been to his recovery. His adventures on the golf course are a testament to all that life is truly worth living, regardless of one's physical limitations.

Jeff's playing partners now hold the flagstick for him.

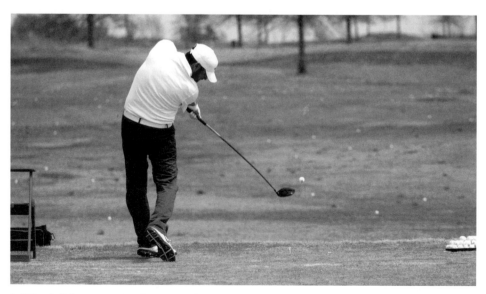

Jeff Bardell demonstrating his swing. (Picture courtesy of Jeff Bardell)

The Orange Lightning Bolt
"'Mr. Determination' reverses the Bolt in the burn unit and rehab center."

John was an ambidextrous golfer growing up in Silver Spring, Maryland. He even had the rare privilege of carrying a three handicap while playing on the Eastern Junior High School boys' six-person golf team. I met John when he was in his late 40s, while he was coordinating his first National Amputee Golf Association's First Swing Golf Clinic. It was there that I learned he had undergone 109 surgical procedures spanning nearly ten years, and was lucky to even be alive.

John had worked for a local Florida power company as a linesman, upgrading equipment in the Palm Beach area of South Florida. In late 1989, he had scaled a 40-foot pole in his belt and spikes, as it was inaccessible via a power lift. As he was retrofitting the line, he was electrocuted! After being rushed to the local hospital, John was airlifted to Jackson Memorial Hospital Burn Center in Miami. The doctors put John into a medically-induced coma for about three months to help with the swelling and pressure on the brain, not to mention the pain caused by burns over 70 percent of his 6'3" body.

While John was in the coma, doctors amputated his left arm and shoulder due to gangrene and the severity of the electrical currents that went through his body.

When John awakened, he spent another two months in the burn unit. This is when John found out that he probably would not speak again since his vocal cords had been badly burned, and that he would not walk again. This was indeed the most difficult and life-changing time of his life, and John recalls the importance of his support system which helped him get through some of the most arduous moments he can remember.

After five months in the burn unit, he was transferred to a rehabilitation center. One Sunday afternoon while he was watching a great golf match on television, his recreational therapist walked into the room. "Oh, so you like golf?" she observed. "Listen, when you're ready you can do it — golf — it can be done." John looked at her and thought, "Yeah, right. I'm missing my left arm and shoulder, I can hardly talk and walk and you think I will be playing golf again?" The way he felt and looked, he could only think that seeing a golf course, let alone playing on one again, was less likely than winning the lottery.

He did, however, tuck her comment of hope under his pillow and flirted with it every now and then. He never forgot his therapist's short simple message.

Coincidentally, right around the same time, his two daughters decided to bring the golf course to the hospital for John for the holiday season. Throughout the long, frustrating and tiring days of recovery, John lay in bed playing the Sega video golf game his older daughter had presented to him. He also kept a firm, one-handed grip on the golf club his younger daughter had purchased in a starter set. John started to feel comfortable holding that club in his right hand throughout the remainder of his hospital stay.

When he was released from the hospital, John went to stay with his sister and family in Valdosta, Georgia. It was there that he met his full-time aid, who continued working John's rehab, rebuilding his strength while awaiting improvement in his blood levels in anticipation of additional surgeries needed to mend his body.

John starting putting on the beige living room carpet daily while befriending the hemi-walker that assisted him as he relearned how to walk short distances again, challenging his balancing issues and his drop foot on his right side, a result of the electricity "blow out" of his right hamstring.

Every time he walked by the living room sliding glass door, he would stare out into the backyard, thinking what it would be like to swing the pitching wedge his neighbor had once given to him.

One cloudy morning, John worked his way out to the well-groomed, fenced backyard, leaned against his wheelchair and swung the club with his right arm. What a great feeling! He repeated this drill for about a month until he felt confident that he would not fall over.

"I think I'm ready to go to the golf course," John said. His aid was right there supporting him, from getting out the front door of the house, to the golf course and back home again. John rented a set of clubs and maneuvered himself around the golf course in a four-wheeled scooter. Using the raised seat that swiveled and helped provide a makeshift standing position, he played golf again for the first time in almost 20 years — and it was terrific! He felt he was watching a shadow of his former self.

Golf gave John the incentive and motivation to move out of his wheelchair and helped in his "spiritual, emotional, physical and mental recovery." Each time he returned to the hospital for additional surgeries, golf was his motivator. He thought of his surgeries as continuous hurdles on an endless track! As the anesthesiologist coached John to count down toward yet another medically-induced round of unconsciousness, John said, "I always held onto golf as long as I could before I went under."

"Golf got me out of a shell and back into life. I suffered deep depression because of my horrific accident, injuries, and surgeries. Golf became a great reason to get out of the hospital, and out of the house and it helped me find balance and strength after each surgery.

"I found talking to others out on the golf course lifted my spirits. It was interesting to watch the expressions of others when they realized they had to play with me. They took one look at me and said 'Oh, boy.' It was even more interesting to watch their expressions when I hit the ball straighter than they did, with only one arm."

Just about everyone asked the same two questions of him: "What happened?" and, "What's with the orange lightning bolt on his golf bag?" John explains that the lightning bolt is there "to remind me that — in a flash — how fast life can change. The walls come down between all of us and before you know it, either swinging one-armed or two-armed, we are all playing the same game."

Eventually John worked up his courage and played in his first of many future tournaments with the National Amputee Golf Association and the North American One-Armed Golfers Association. He saw other amputees playing golf and said, "If they can do it, so can I." At these events, John felt he was able to share and enjoy camaraderie and competition.

"Golf does so much for your inner peace and confidence. Golf is my church with God and nature. Golf seems to have it all for me." With scars as thick as cables under his arm, he shares that in spite of having the phantom sensation, he still remembers what it is like to set up to the ball with two arms and can still feel his left hand on the club before he draws his backswing. "I may not have a left arm to push or pull the club, but I do hit it straighter with just one arm."

Because of what the golf did for him, John decided to become an ambassador to the game by serving as a board member for the North American One Armed Golf Association in the early 2000s. His mission is to encourage individuals to respect the golf course and other players, as well as educate inquiring minds when they ask about "our injuries."

"Tell them and educate them," he says. John feels very strongly that because of the game of golf and his tremendous support system of loved ones, friends, neighbors, therapists and doctors who told him never to give up, he has achieved his goal of recovery.

John told his foursome at the end of the round one day, "If golf helped me through my recovery, and it got me to this point in my life after what I went through, it can help others."

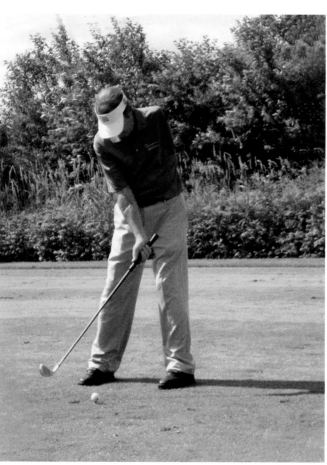

John Barton with a one-armed set up. (Picture courtesy of John Barton)

Trading in Hardwood Floors for the Green Carpet

"I have this huge world in front of me and in a matter of a few seconds I have narrowed down life to a tiny little white ball. It's yoga-like."

A well-spoken man in his mid-forties rolled his wheelchair into one of the hitting stations where I was teaching during an accessible golf clinic at a well kept golf course in Tampa, Florida. An ad in the local newspaper had caught Cliff's attention. A veteran wheelchair basketball player, he was pondering what to do after retiring from bouncing an orange and black ball up and down the hardwood floors.

Like all serious competitive athletes, Cliff was in search of the next recreational activity, or substitute, to fulfill his adrenaline rush. Other athletes traded in footballs pads, hockey sticks, tennis racquets and baseball bats. Cliff would be trading in his basketball and jersey for a bag of graphite sticks — his new recreational vehicle of amusement.

The game of golf is like a magnet, attracting participants from all generations, from professional athlete and amateur, to housewife and entrepreneur.

Golf is one of the most sought after games and "conversion" sports there is. It is the easiest, yet hardest — yes, I said that — the easiest, yet hardest sport I know. And it is golf's rules of engagement that enable it to be accessible to anyone.

Cliff, a First Lieutenant with the U.S. Army, had served for six years, including a stint in Desert Storm, before a 1991 automobile accident stateside left him a "super quad."

Though he'd rarely played golf in his younger days, he had always been intrigued by the game. An avid tennis and basketball player prior to enlisting, it seemed appropriate that his sport of choice post-paralysis became wheelchair basketball in the National Wheelchair Basketball League. He loved the competition and camaraderie.

On that brilliant sunny autumn day, Cliff applied the hand brakes to his wheelchair and shared with me that he played guard for one of the 150 wheelchair basketball teams that traveled around the country. You cannot play wheelchair basketball, maneuvering a two-wheeled seat around a court with nine other men chasing and shooting a ball, if you do not have great chair skills. I quickly gathered that Cliff was an extremely coordinated individual. Though not a requirement, this coordination was an added bonus for making contact with the tiny ball.

Due to some pressure sores, Cliff was currently on injured reserve, which really hit me. Isn't it difficult enough to be paralyzed, without having to be out on "injured reserve" added to it? Where is the fairness in that? As we continued to talk, it became increasingly apparent to me that wheelchair basketball and golf have much in common. Cliff's background of hard work, dedication and a strong work ethic coupled with his athletic build were only going to compliment his golfing experiences.

When it comes to teaching golf to the physically challenged, there is no one best position or right way to swing a club because of the differences of severities associated with each injury. Since Cliff has a C-5 functional spinal cord injury, we explored a handful of different approaches. What came most naturally to him was swinging in his own chair with a special club bent 15 degrees flat. His wheelchair was positioned to an "open stance" in relationship to the target line.

He placed his left hand on the wheelchair for support, similar to negotiating his chair around the basketball court for stability and direction. Then he swung at the ball effortlessly with his right arm, approximating a rebound, pass or shot in a basketball game. With consistency he hit the ball 60-70 yards in the air, down the middle of the driving range. Not bad for a man who couldn't use his legs!

Cliff's smile grew as wide as the range. "This is pretty easy," he said, a feeling of confidence and happiness bursting from him. What I remembered most about Cliff was that he had little to no expectations, which led to a contentment of outcome. I silently wondered why more able-bodied golfers couldn't carry a more light hearted approach to their game.

Too many golfers become bogged down with technical thoughts as they try to swing the club back and forth, or as I call it "connecting-the-dots." They become so mechanical and "positional" that nothing moves freely. I found it interesting that Cliff did not ask me if he was starting the club back correctly or if his club was in the right position at the top of his back swing, as most able-bodied players do.

He just imitated my motion and swung through the ball. Obviously, less is more. In Cliff's case, he had fewer moving parts rotating over a stable foundation, and he was able to connect consistently with the ball.

Cliff declared, "Golf has done wonders for my focus on the court, especially my free throw. Golf to me is very relaxing. I have this huge world in front of me and in a matter of seconds I have to narrow down life to a tiny little white ball. It's yoga-like."

At a picnic table with some of his fellow vets, Cliff shared his thoughts on golf and the clinic. "This is a great stepping stone to get started, or re-enter life. The next time you are lying in bed beating yourself up, get out to a golf course or driving range immediately. It's good to get outside in the fresh air." He added, "Today has been extra special for me because I got to socialize, meet new people and see my old basketball buddies."

I think we did our job of hooking Cliff on the game played on the green carpet. He demonstrated his ability and expertise in his newly-discovered sport, sharing his exuberance, joy and gratitude with colleagues. Cliff is well on his way to rolling into a new-found passion once his days on the court have ended. ⛳

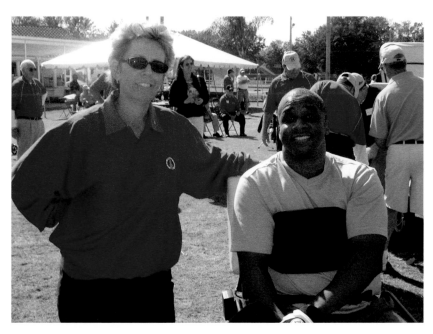

Cliff's smile says it all.

An Interesting Twist of Fate

"Even with one arm, you can score a hole-in-one."

In the summer of 1994, I teed it up with Gail, a very pleasant and dynamic woman and co-founder of RE/MAX, LLC. We teamed together in a golf tournament in Denver, conducted by the Association of Disabled American Golfers.

Eleven years earlier, and one month prior to Gail marrying Dave Liniger, the love of her life, a near-fatal small plane crash left her paralyzed. As a result of a traumatic brain injury, Gail was unable to move her left side. Their date to meet at the altar was postponed. Over that long winter, Gail regained her strength and the following spring she and Dave were married.

I was mesmerized by how Gail, a right-sided one-armed golfer, maneuvered around the hilly golf course and demonstrated incredible perseverance. Although she limped and moved more slowly than the average golfer, Gail acknowledged how much the game helped her health, strength and personal fitness.

She immediately understood the benefits of golf: "I can play this game forever. Dave and I play whenever we travel; age and location are never a barrier. When I am on the golf course, I am totally relaxed, leaving all office worries behind." She added, "Even with one arm, you can score a hole-in-one." She should know. She's done it.

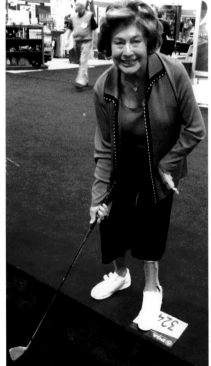

Since her recovery, Gail and Dave have encouraged many charities to utilize The Sanctuary Golf Course, their privately owned course in Sedalia, for fundraising events. Since 1997, a total of $56 million has been raised by 284 charitable events conducted at their breathtaking golf course. Gail and Dave have been honored with prestigious awards for their generous philanthropy.

Gail demonstrating her set-up.

Because Dave is an Air Force veteran of the Vietnam War, the Linigers also provide assistance to organizations that support our troops, including the Sentinels of Freedom Foundation. Its mission is to provide men and women of the U.S. Armed Forces who have suffered severe injuries up to a four-year "life scholarship" toward self-sufficiency.

Additionally, the Sanctuary Golf Course sponsors Military Days, when members of the Army, Air Force, and Marines are invited out on their respective service day for a complimentary round of golf. These are two incredibly generous people. Gail's recovery and resiliency are inspiring, Dave's support unwavering. They chose to put a positive spin on a twist of fate, and have both given so much to so many through the game of golf.

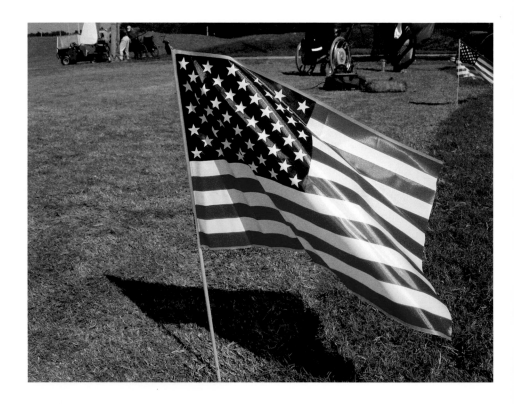

The Back Nine

Golf Through the Darkness
"I realized playing golf is about trusting yourself."

Every weekend golf enthusiasts of all ages turn on the TV to watch the greatest ball-strikers in the world tee it up, hoping their favorite player will walk down the 18th hole on Sunday and claim victory. Each player is surrounded by their "team" of experts: caddie, personal trainer, swing coach, mental coach, nutritionist, agent; and the list goes on. Each team could form their own gallery!

But what about those who face insurmountable odds and who do not have a "team" of experts in their corner? What happens to those with a team of one? And, what happens when that one person, the "coach" has to actually become the player's eyes — because the golfer is blind? Well, that one person is quite possibly far more important than any member of any entourage of any tour player. That's what Tina is — she is Bob's wife/coach.

Bob Andrews is a blind golfer with an enviable swing who hits the ball better than most weekend hackers. But Bob needs what they call a "coach," and that's where Tina comes into play. I call the twosome the "true love team."

Bob, a young Marine, was falling in love with Tina when he pushed off to serve in Vietnam.

Before he left, he had asked her to marry him upon his return from Vietnam — she said yes. While fighting for our freedom, Bob sustained multiple injuries including losing his sight to shrapnel from a grenade blast that nearly killed him. The tough Marine fought valiantly and returned to the United States to start a new chapter in his life, which included marrying Tina. While recovering in the VA hospital, Bob was introduced to the game of golf through the blind rehabilitation program. He embraced it to the point that he ultimately became the president of the United States Blind Golf Association.

Our paths crossed many years ago in Myrtle Beach, South Carolina, where we were both attending a National Forum on Accessible Golf. I was paired with Bob and Tina at a golf outing. Running a little late to the first tee, I met them on the approach shots to the first green. I had never experienced playing golf with a blind golfer; as a golf instructor, I was looking forward to the experience. I was just really curious how he was going to play golf when he couldn't see. I mean come on — we use our eyes for everything, or so I thought! Little did I know.

How is it possible for the blind or visually-impaired golfer to "see" the golf course? To play a round of golf? Aren't they just as constricted by missing the beauty our game has to offer?

Close your eyes for a minute. Go ahead. What do you see? Black? Purple? Yellow? Now, imagine playing 18 holes like that.

Bob and Tina told me to go ahead and hit, so I dropped a ball in the fairway, threw some grass up into the air to get a read on the wind, figured out my yardage, selected my stick, lined up my shot and put the ball on the green.

Across the fairway, Bob and Tina were orchestrating their "team work." I could see the "oneness" that existed between the two of them. She gave the yardage, the direction and the condition of the lie. He pointed his face towards the sky and turned it from side to side to feel the wind with his face and body. He said, "Let me have my 7-iron." She placed the grip end in between his hands. After he took a few practice swings, she placed the club head right behind the ball and aligned him up to the center of the green. She moved over and said "clear" indicating it was safe for him to swing.

With a very neat, organized and balanced swing, the ball flew gracefully into the air and landed some 20 feet past the cup. It was amazing to watch him feel his swing and absorb the shot. Tina walked him back to the cart and they drove toward the green.

I wondered if Bob was the one who had an advantage over me. He never saw the low to high parking-lot sized green surrounded by large white sandy bunkers on either side with a body of water in front. What fascinated me the most was that Tina never even told him about the water and the bunkers. When you think about it, he didn't need to know. He just lined up and swung freely as if he was on automatic-pilot.

I got to thinking that all golfers should swing more freely, like Bob. Stop steering and controlling, just let it happen by simply feeling the shot. That is exactly what Bob was doing. Since he couldn't see, he had to rely on his other senses. He had to have the epitome of trust in his "coach" and be able to feel the club going back and forth. He had to feel the swinging motion and listen for significant sounds that sighted golfers miss in the game.

These sounds are important to Bob, like the sound of the ball colliding with the driver as he crushed the ball down the middle of the fairway.

Bob listened as an iron swept through the grass blades in a practice swing; he listened to the swoosh sound as the club swung back and forth with his body. And, the best sound of all, when his ball dropped into the cup. It clanked and swirled around before settling to the bottom. He liked this sound most of all. Too bad all those people who take "gimmes" don't hear this wonderful sound!

Sometimes seeing less in our sport is more. I think most sighted golfers refuse to see what the golf course has to offer. They only see the trouble and the doom and gloom that await their shot. As an instructor, I'm always wondering what's going on inside my student's head as they get ready to swing and strike the ball. Are they thinking positively or actually sabotaging themselves? Are they confident or fearful? Next time you're on the course, ask yourself these questions and then think of the shots from Bob's point of view.

Bob demonstrated to me that we can play the game of golf whether our vision works or not. We don't need all of our sight to feel our way around a golf course.

We could all learn from Bob by not reading too much into what we see on the golf course. We should learn from Bob that he was in control of his game and not the other way around. We should trust our "coach" and allow them to be our windows to a golf course.

Playing with Bob made me realize that there is much to see on a golf course. I wish others had the opportunity to see what this blind man "can see."

It is amazing how our eyes are the windows to the world and how much we take for granted. I was so fortunate to witness true love on the course. I realized playing golf is about trusting yourself and your surroundings; like swinging naked. Thank you, Bob and Tina, for allowing me to see beyond my eyes in this wonderful game of golf. ◉

When Push Comes to Shove

"You really can do anything if you put your mind to it."

Three of them came rolling at me, arms pumping their wheelchairs and pointing their forefingers in synch. "We need you." It was as if an Uncle Sam recruiting poster had come to life. I turned to look behind me because I knew they weren't . . . nah, they couldn't be talking to me. Sure enough, they were.

They needed a fourth to fill one side in an eight-person wheelchair basketball pick-up game. So, like a reserve coming off the bench, I hustled. I ran down the bleachers, hurtling over

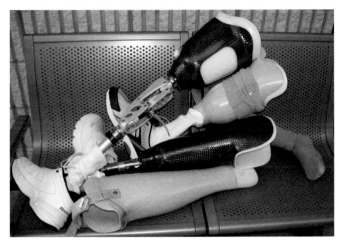

a pile of prosthetic legs. The eager team helped me strap my two legs into an amazingly colorful high-tech sports wheelchair. My heart was pounding. What an adrenaline rush! The thought of playing basketball with these guys was certainly unique to me as I'd never done anything like this before. I've played basketball, but not from a seated position. Without legs, the challenge was daunting.

Just moments earlier I'd been semi-daydreaming, catching up on some e-mails and returning phone calls. I had tucked myself high up in the corner of the metal bleachers of a very bright indoor basketball court waiting to catch a red-eye back to the east coast.

The pick-up game was taking place at the Naval Medical Center San Diego in California. I'd been in town for 48 hours, training several golf professionals called upon to teach the game to the men and women returning from Operation Enduring Freedom and Operation Iraqi Freedom, as well as other combat theaters.

When I awakened that day, it never occurred to me that I would be getting a "crash" course — literally, as wheelchairs collided with each other like bumper cars — on playing wheelchair basketball from some of the bravest men who had gone to war to protect my country's freedom.

In that game, I was transformed from being their golf instructor earlier in the day to serving as an "official fill-in sub" at night. I had no idea how hard this was going to be. I was breathless; my fingers became entangled in the spokes of the chair as I attempted to alter my direction and speed. Coordination became paramount. The art of maneuvering a wheelchair while playing basketball was just as difficult as playing golf blindfolded. Halfway through the game, the other end of the court started looking as far away as a marathon finish line.

All these strong men became my teachers, giving me advice on how to "Push the wheelchair like this", "Stop and turn like this!" "Speed up this way and slow down this way." "Shoot! Block!" With all these tips on how to roll the chair, get the ball, block the shot, or steal the ball, I was reminded just what my golf students go through when they are trying to learn something new or different.

Making five birdies in a row seemed easier than attempting a free throw from a seated position. I just didn't have the upper body strength to throw it that high and far. Yet I wanted to impress the guys. They had come out to the golf course earlier in the day exposing their vulnerabilities; the least I could do was show them the same respect.

Sitting in that wheelchair, trying to keep up with these men who had been involved in wheelchair basketball for a few years since losing either one or both legs to IED's was one of the special adventures of my life.

I was reminded just how powerful golf is to someone in recovery. It underscores the essence of staying active to someone who has lost a part of his or her body and is forever a changed person.

As we rolled over to the sideline, I had a reality check. I simply got up and out of the chair; I didn't have to reattach one or two prosthetic legs first. This was a profound reminder to be thankful for what I have in my life. I embraced this life lesson as I flew home that night.

Although my team lost the game that evening, I affirmed a renewed sense that when push comes to shove, you really CAN do anything if you put your mind to it. Just ask the guys in the chairs!

Moment of "Impact"

"The look on his face was incredible! He pulled his shoulder blades back, pushed his chest forward and painted on a smile as wide as the Pacific Ocean."

When someone is striking golf balls, whether from a seated or standing position, on one leg or with one arm, it is amazing to witness just one crowd pleasing shot. You know that clean powerful sound that leaves a profound effect and an indelible mental image. You can hear the "crack" and virtually feel the impact.

One crisp spring day, I was conducting an accessible golf training session for PGA Professionals at a golf course in the Mission Gorge area of San Diego. A subdued young lieutenant named Tim Jeffers volunteered to be our "student" on the driving range for the afternoon session. He wasn't your typical student. Four months earlier, as a result of injuries sustained from an IED in Iraq, he lost both legs just above the knees as well as his right ring finger, and was wearing a TBI helmet protecting his head following cranial reconstructive surgery.

Other than hitting a few balls with his buddies when he was in high school, Tim was inexperienced and, needless to say, rather nervous. Add to the fact that there were 20 people standing in a semi-circle preparing to watch him receive his first golf lesson.

After introductions we shared with Tim — who was strapped into a single-rider cart — that we were going to show him a variety of swing techniques with different clubs to get an idea of what he could handle. At first, Tim was whiffing, and then topping the ball, becoming a bit frustrated with each missed opportunity. But that didn't last too long due to our host, PGA Professional John Klein, who owns one of the largest smorgasbord and heaviest golf bag of adaptive clubs I had ever seen. We experimented, narrowing down the best club for Tim to use swinging from a seated position. Many misses and topped shots later he started connecting with the ball. The look on his face was incredible! Tim pulled his shoulder blades back, pushed his chest forward and painted on a smile as wide as the Pacific Ocean. There was such a strong sense of accomplishment and confidence exuding from this wounded warrior, which was much greater than most of the golf professionals in the audience could fathom. Launching the golf ball into the air had created an awesome feeling for this proud Marine.

This, of course, is but one shining example of the significant "impact" the game of golf can have on a wounded warrior.

"It is a transformation of spirit that overcomes the student as much as us, their instructors," said a PGA Professional. Klein was overheard saying, "By keeping it simple and working with his ability, we created a golf swing to give him a new reason to have fun."

Following the clinic, this successful warrior shared with us, "I'm glad I volunteered. I was really nervous knowing everyone would be looking at me but getting out in the fresh air, compared to being stuck in that rehab center, showed me that I could do something without my legs."

 He felt good about it! That day, on that range, we shared. The teachable moments were reciprocal; we reached a new level of achievement, not measured in feet or yards, but in the freedom of movement and recognition of new milestones. The impact on each of us was most profound.

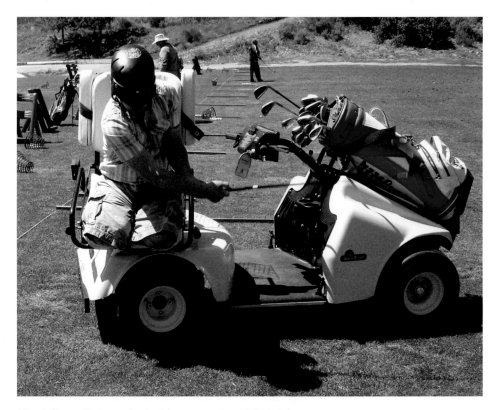

Tim Jeffers utilizing a single rider cart and modified clubs.

From Concrete Hallways to Green Fairways
"It's nice to be out of the hospital for the day in the fresh air."

VA hospitals. What do you think of when you hear those words? I used to think of concrete buildings, endless paperwork, patients taking a number, getting lost in the shuffle, thinking, "I fought for my country and this is how I am treated?" I thought of a broken system in need of help . . . and hopefully a means to an end. Now, when I hear the words "VA hospital," I am reminded of the time I participated as a trainer and instructor for the American Veterans Accessible Golf Program, a two-day seminar in Tampa, Florida run, by PGA Professional David Windsor.

Admittedly, I was somewhat nervous, not knowing where I was going or what to expect. Fighting early morning traffic and construction in the hospital parking lot did not help! However, that was nothing compared to trying to find the room where we were holding our seminar. I guess now I know what a golfer goes through when they visit my facility for the first time. The fear of the unknown, and wondering how to get from point A to point B.

Walking through this massive building, searching for the seminar was like trying to find that proverbial hole-in-one. I found myself on an endless journey of mazes through dimly lit corridors, with signs on walls with arrows pointing this way and that, up a flight of stairs, and then an elevator to a particular floor. Before I knew it I was in an overcrowded waiting room, unfortunately at the wrong end of the hospital. I made a U-turn, asked for directions, and realized this place was dauntingly huge.

During this search for the seminar room I kept comparing this isolated walk to one down the lush green fairways of an aesthetically appealing golf course. There was also a second thought that entered my mind — I am making this hike on my own two legs. I couldn't possibly imagine pushing myself in a wheelchair or using crutches to carry out this seemingly endless search. As I walked the hallways I passed many people and wondered whether they were hurt in current or previous combat theaters and how they were coping. Were their situations temporary or life changing? Wow! Golf courses are so much more tranquil, hospitable, picturesque and soothing.

FINALLY . . . I discovered the right room and took my seat among the audience. I almost felt out of place, as this scenery wasn't what I was accustomed to on a golf course or in everyday life. I was surrounded by so many patients missing limbs, in different phases of their rehab, on crutches or standing on prosthetics of all technological phases. One young man was even wearing a helmet. Some were lying on gurneys wheeled in for this occasion, with pins and rods protruding from different body parts, gauze tape, ace bandages and IVs hanging on poles shadowing their owners.

The room included both active and retired military and medical personnel. I must have resembled an emotional rainbow with colors of excitement, nervousness and fear; however, I realized we were all gathered in this place because of one common link, the game of golf.

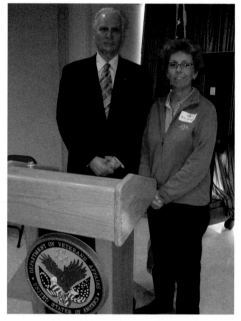

As I settled into my seat to listen to the tall distinguished guest speaker, I felt suddenly overwhelmed. It was as if I had been hit by a stun gun. Our speaker, Captain George Burk, USAF (Ret. Vietnam veteran), described in great detail his near-death experience as the sole survivor of 14 passengers in a military plane crash, leaving him with burns over 65 percent of his body and multiple internal injuries.

Captain George Burk, USAF and Judy Alvarez.

He went on to say that he spent 90 days in ICU and 18 months in the hospital. This was beyond my personal comprehension. I was amazed by how much a human body can endure physically, emotionally, mentally, and still survive. He stressed to the survivors in the audience, "You will get through this phase of your life. You will move on. Look at what I overcame." The audience was silent.

Each of us was moved by his inspirational message of having faith and overcoming adversity, conveying the will to survive, persevere and never give up. I fought back tears. Who wouldn't after listening to a passionate message like this? I have never been on the front line of combat, nor do I know what it is like to have a life-changing injury, but I do know just how intoxicating the game of golf can be to the wounded warriors. When I think about it,

I get a feeling in the pit of my stomach that I do not get from reading any golf manuals. I knew beyond a doubt that the golf therapy program these military men and women would be exposed to over the next two days was going to be wonderful for them. They just didn't know it yet!

Later that day, under a clear blue sky with white cotton clouds, volunteers, golf professionals and therapists were busy setting up the driving range for an expected attendance of more than 80 people. As the hitting stations began to fill to capacity with veterans of current and previous combat theaters and their loved ones, each station had its own unique story. One retired vet was a BK (below knee) amputee, while another station was occupied by a paraplegic hitting balls from a seated electric golf cart. Next to him was a tall, slender young man standing on two legs, swinging with only his left arm. To the east of him was a lefty swinging with his right arm. Holding down another station was a paunchy man who was an AK (above knee) amputee; he was so proud to be a Marine that he had the Seal of the United States Marine Corps tattooed on the calf side of his prosthetic. Some vets were wearing advanced high technology prosthetics, while others were bearing older conventional ones that were not as maneuverable.

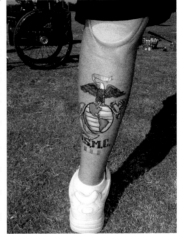

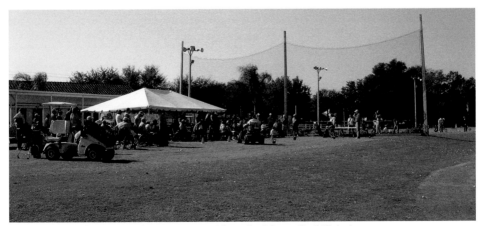

A perfect day of inclusion. (participants with and without disabilities)

On any given day, as golf instructors, we will diagnose a variety of typical different swing flaws and prescribe the correct remedy, but on this day, each vet brought with them their own unique set of abilities and we had to adapt quickly with outside-the-box thinking.

Our duty was to listen and support the players — not try to fix them. After winding through so many grim concrete corridors earlier in the day, I saw just how important being outside on a practice range could truly be to a wounded warrior. Fresh air, sunshine, blue skies, bonding, socializing, laughing, joking, sharing funny stories, eating a meal "off base" and being with loved ones, or even making new friends created this "healing the soul" environment.

I knew we had done our job when I heard comments like:

> "This was a great day."
>
> "We had so much fun!"
>
> "It was good to talk to other vets."
>
> "It was so nice to be outside."
>
> "It was so nice to get out of the hospital."
>
> "It was cool to take a whack at the ball!"

Funny how their view is so different from ours. A day outside in the sunshine is better than any day confined to a VA hospital bed. Being in an environment where the possibility presents itself to hit balls and enjoy the moment is far healthier than being depressed inside. I must always remind myself, it's not the flight of the ball and the score that matters as much as providing an uplifting experience.

As we were wrapping up the day, these great warriors took a moment to say, "Thanks for all that you do." They were so appreciative that we took time out of our lives to help them. At that moment I wondered who was giving to whom? It reminded me not to take the game of golf for granted and to look for the camouflaged intangibles the game has to offer: it can truly be a foundation for someone to recover and grow and heal.

Suffice it to say, our "safe, nothing blows up" battlefield of golf carts, buckets of balls and golf clubs provided a fun atmosphere for these brave men and women and their families. It was certainly safer than the battlefields they had fought on to defend our country. My gratitude and thanks goes out to all of them. ⛳

Golf: One Link in the Care Chain

"Since losing my leg, golf has been one of the most vital forms of therapy."

I snapped my head when I heard the sound of the ball ripping off the clubface. That booming sound always gets me, especially when it echoes under a covered driving range. The striped ball propelled a good 230 yards straight down the middle of the muddy range. Compelled to see who was swinging the club, I meandered closer to see that the man responsible for flattening the dimples on the golf ball was doing it on one leg.

Yes, that's right, on one leg and he wasn't using a crutch as support. As a matter of fact, his crutches were leaning up against the green stall metal divider and, as I found out later, his prosthetic leg was in his house. He literally was crushing balls balanced on his left leg. His right leg was somewhere in the hot arid sand overseas, blown away by a 120 mm mortar round in 2005, when he served in the military, defending our country's freedom.

The game of golf and Chief Warrant Officer Daniel Parker didn't meet eye-to-eye for quite some time. Like so many people, this average size man with chocolate brown eyes thought golf was one of those "stupid" sports. After all, he had been a baseball and hockey player prior to enlisting and that all changed in a flash.

I first met Dan, a bald man from Nebraska, while he was going through rehab at Walter Reed Army Medical Center in Washington. I was in our nation's capital training PGA Professionals in the Middle Atlantic PGA Section. These professionals would be teaching a military accessible golf program for wounded warriors, headed by the on-site PGA Golf Professional, Jim Estes, at Olney Golf Park, and sponsored in part by Disabled Sports USA.

Like so many veterans returning from Iraq, this "Cornhusker" was dealing with a list of emotions: grief, depression, despair and hopelessness brought on by losing his leg, fighting for his life, enduring nightmares of his buddies dying in the explosion, and having to relearn some of the most basic necessities of life. For Dan, each day seemed overwhelming.

Characteristic of many vets, Dan questioned which direction his life was headed, especially since returning dismembered. He went overseas with two legs and returned with far less. He was grieving. From this point forward life would be different. Battling rehab day after day, week after week, attempting to get better while watching others go through the same issues, was taking a toll on him.

After resisting countless offers and advice to get "off campus" for at least one day a week, Dan finally caved in and said he would give it a try. He realized that becoming involved in some form of physical activity would be both therapeutic and healing. Golf became an immediate attraction.

Since Dan was an amputee— better known as an AK (above the knee) it was difficult to wear his prosthetic socket over his stump and hip while swinging because it restricted his hip from effectively rotating like a golfer's. So, in the early stages of learning to play golf, he removed his prosthetic, tossed it on the ground and like many others, he never looked back. Instead, he learned how to hit balls on one leg. Granted, success wasn't coming at a fast enough pace for this proud father; he was determined to be good at what he was doing and as it turned out, he "kind of enjoyed it." I couldn't help but wonder how he didn't fall over hitting golf balls for hours and hours on one leg, but this man has impeccable balance.

Determined to hit on his left leg and not use his prosthetic, his golf instructor, Jim Estes, capitalized on this vet's above-average balance by giving him some additional balancing drills to build up his stamina, keeping in mind that fatigue was certainly an inhibiting factor in the beginning. Jim suggested some drills, like he does to many other vets:

- Work up to standing on one leg with eyes closed for up to one minute
- Work up to hitting balls for 30 minutes

Between private lessons and group golf classes, balance exercises and ball striking, Dan's attitude improved. The word "can't" was replaced with "how can I?" He went on to say, "This sport looks so easy. Well, until you try it, you just don't know how physically demanding the sport is," which was pretty impressive coming from a former baseball and hockey player!

The honored vet said, "Since losing my leg, golf has been one of the most vital forms of therapy. It was a way to rebuild my confidence in my physical appearance and it was a great physical activity." Even if someone else couldn't tell Dan was an amputee, it was painfully obvious to him.

When people ask me how a golf instructor can help men and women like Dan, I tell them this vet's story is very similar to others I've met over the years. To me, it is the definition of what it means to be a golf instructor.

Exposing Dan to the game of golf was like giving him a ladder to climb out of his depression, escape the enclosures of Walter Reed, and provide opportunities to meet new people whom he now cherishes as best friends.

Dan has learned the meaning of time shared with friends hitting balls on the driving range. People, who have shared such a traumatic experience together, as these many men did in Iraq, can look at each other and express, without saying anything, "I know. I was there with you. It's OK." So if they hit good shots they were happy and if they hit bad shots, they didn't care. Golf has taught them to just have fun.

Dan like so many others said, "The driving range is another great place to test yourself." And when asked if he would encourage other vets to play golf, he answered, "Oh yea. Definitely! This range is a BIG confidence-builder for me. Maybe your body doesn't look and work the same, and you may not be good in the beginning but you will be if you stick with it." Isn't that a legitimate statement of all of life's challenges? Or, is it not true of everything that life throws at us?

Subsequently, Dan realized he could spend his time not only helping himself but also others who were going through similar life changes. He realized that even though he had lost his leg, there was someone who was worse off and could use his help. Going to golf class was another way of getting involved and a way to give back to others who were new at their recovery.

Eventually bombing golf balls some 220 yards became routine for Dan. No more sitting in rehab feeling sorry for himself or self-medicating or drinking to forget life's worries. Golf or self-medicating? Hmm! Seems like an obvious choice to me and an excellent choice for Dan!

Apparently the challenge this "stupid" sport presented to Dan paid off. His mobility and self-confidence increased. He realized that if he could hit balls off one leg, he could also excel in other aspects of his life. If he survived the hot, arid war zone, he could overcome learning a new sport.

More and more, critics like Dan, who have suffered an injury are giving the game a try and realizing that it's not easy. They embrace the challenge and they do not give up.

I am not sure if Dan knows how much he has touched me, as a golf instructor, and I want to thank him for that. It is just so extraordinary and wonderful to see Dan hit great golf shots off one leg. I'm not sure if my able-bodied students, or "normies," will like this, but the "Dans" of the world have made me a better instructor.

Here's the reality of it: First, if Dan can hit balls off one leg, shouldn't someone with two legs be able to hit a ball successfully? It reinforced the importance of having a positive attitude when learning something new. I call it "purging"— getting rid of all that extra useless garbage a golfer carries around with them. He also demonstrated again to me as an instructor how important balance and staying centered over the ball are during a swing.

Second, I have carried Dan's healing story with me during my training sessions and shared with other golf professionals the importance of including wounded warriors and the injured in golf programs.

Third, it's neat to know that Dan has been converted to a golfer who now has profound respect for golf as a recreational sport.

Lastly, what I take to heart the most are people who are willing to take chances with their lives. Dan did. He tried something new and different. It changed the course of his recovery, which has given hope to others who are in situations similar to his.

It turns out that Dan liked the challenge and now he is a golf addict. He joined the golf program at the local park and has since learned the true essence of what golf really means. Golf has given him a life outside the military.

I thank Jim and other golf instructors and friends for providing a circle of support and generosity of spirit that has encouraged Dan, and so many others, to see there is so very much life has to offer after a life-changing experience, and, that golf is a joyful, healthy, wonderful transition from battlefield to civilian life.

A Fairway for Us to Give Back

"I don't care about your opinion on war. Support the cause?
Maybe or maybe not. Support the person? Absolutely."

One chilly spring morning in Washington DC a military vet placed red carnations atop the white marble headstone of his fallen friend. As the bright sun glared on the morning dew, I stood there watching his penetrating eyes and wondered what he was really looking at and thinking about. Was he having a silent conversation with his friend? When he gave the smart and snappy military salute to his buddy and it wasn't returned, it sent shivers down my spine as I stood in the background. Although it was a quiet morning, the silence was incredibly deafening.

Later that day, as I watched the Army sharpshooter hit golf balls, I kept wondering what had been behind that stare of his? Was it touchable? Would he share with me? Could I truly see the windows to his soul? I can gaze into his eyes all I want and will never truly know what he experienced. He fought for my country's freedom at the cost of losing a limb and returned with invisible battle scars. I did not serve in the military; I have absolutely no idea what it is like to aim a gun and shoot at the enemy.

What is it like living with indelible pictures etched in your memory? Can I have an impact on these battle-weary warriors? Can what I, and other golf instructors, offer really change or shape their lives for the better? How can we actually contribute to making a difference?

What can we possibly do to help them and their loved ones after what they've been through? Sometimes I feel helpless — but not hopeless. Rehab teams are comprised of doctors, therapists, prosthetists, family, and friends. Why not add a golf instructor to the team? Since our freedom comes at a cost, the least we can do is take the time to listen, demonstrate compassion, provide lessons and accessible golf programs, offer access to golf courses and tournaments, and provide modified equipment. It doesn't sound difficult.

Perhaps this is how we golf professionals can give back. We can facilitate the process and simplify the procedures. We can be a catalyst for change in the rehabilitation program.

PGA Professional Don Vickery of Savannah, Georgia, served his country from 1976-83 and lost both legs in 1989. As the first double amputee to earn PGA membership, he says,

"Golf pros are always willing to help someone. It's the nature of who we are. We don't want to leave people behind."

Let's use the golf course as a road to recovery, one fairway at a time, one swing at a time. We already have the ball field — we just need to send out the invitation. We have built it — let them come.

Over the years I have had the opportunity to talk to many men and women who have served in the armed forces in current and previous combat theaters. The recurring theme has always been that on a variety of levels, golf is an important therapeutic tool and a saving grace for those who have served us, regardless of when their injury occurred.

It's fascinating that these veterans would make a comment like this about my industry, my career, my passion. It is amazing that 18 holes spread out over roughly 100 acres of green grass can facilitate the transformation of changing and saving lives, snap someone out of depression, lift a spirit and enhance a family nucleus. As a golf professional, I know that we get caught up in the hustle and bustle of the everyday requirements our business demands of us and forget just how powerful a representation our ball field is for our veterans in the face of freedom.

Retired Major Ed Pulido, a Purple Heart recipient from Edmond, Oklahoma, and Senior Vice President of Programs and Veterans Affairs of the Folds of Honor Foundation, lost his left leg in 2004 after an IED explosion in Baqubah, Iraq. He laid out the value of a golf course for wounded warriors.

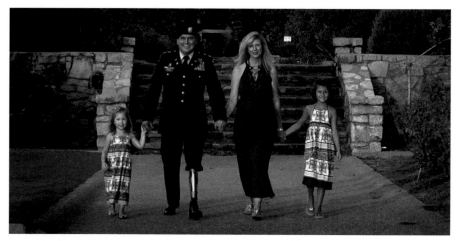

Retired Major Ed Pulido says that he has "healed more quickly because of golf."
(Picture courtesy of Ed Pulido)

"It's a place where they can find out just how good they can be," says this heroic family man. "It's where recovery is possible. You have to grasp it and run with it. It's where hitting the ball right is secondary to hitting it at all." Major Pulido says that he has "healed more quickly because of golf."

I have to agree. I have witnessed the metamorphosis of individuals due to the game of golf. One of the most heart-wrenching comments I have heard in my teaching career was when a solider said, "Thank you for putting on this golf clinic. Lately I've been thinking of committing suicide." The smile on his face at the end of our clinic sent a powerful message, that golf can be a place where troubled souls can be soothed and calmed, that golf is a necessity for our wounded warriors, perhaps maybe even on some levels we cannot comprehend.

In some way, we golf professionals owe the opportunity to restore body and mind through golf to the very souls who voluntarily signed up to defend our country and came back dismembered or permanently scarred. As PGA Professional Doug MacArthur says, "It is an honor to coach our service men and woman, who sacrifice their lives and bodies."

Can you think of any other place to spend time recovering? Major Pulido remarks, "The golfing community can be the backbone of embracing our armed forces. The golf course is a wonderful, beautiful and tranquil outdoor environment."

Think about it: most of these men and women are fighting outdoors in hot, arid, lonely, frightening places. How wonderful for them to be able to transition to our environment, where the worst they have to contend with is a greenside bunker, an encroaching water hazard or a bogey.

Golf is a potent prescription for broken spirits who carry around hidden wounds and have lost their compass on life. Wounded warriors who are introduced to golf can begin to feel better about themselves.

As Vickery said, "Whatever you want to do in life is not up to your injury, it's up to you. Don't let your injury dictate what you can and cannot do in life." When he paid a visit to the vets at Walter Reed Army Medical Center as a kindred spirit, Vickery told many of the vets, "You have to work at it. It's difficult. You will get a greater return out of it the more you work at it. However, you have got to get up and fight through it. Prosthetics are like new shoes; they hurt. It's difficult but not impossible. There is a return. You put the work in and you will get something out of it."

What Vickery describes is the ongoing inherent value of the game of golf. It reflects life's challenges. In fact, they run parallel to one other. You get just as much out of the game of golf — and life — as you put into it.

PGA Professional David Windsor, who runs the Adaptive Golf Academy in Tampa, Florida, echoes Vickery, "For wounded warriors and disabled vets, the game of golf is the best well-rounded recreational therapy. Golf is changing the way they think about themselves, which ultimately improves their lives."

Many vets are fortunate to work on their golf game at Olney Golf Park in Maryland. PGA Professional Jim Estes, a co-founder of Salute Military Golf Association, says, "Many of the golf programs I offer have been a recipe for overall success. Just watching these vets grow day after day and week and after week is wonderful. They need to get out of the VA hospital and come to a golf program to get started. Once they come here, they change."

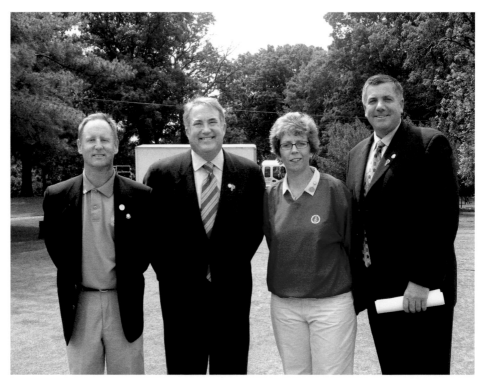

PGA Professional Jim Estes, CEO of PGA of America Joseph Steranka, PGA/LPGA Professional Judy Alvarez, PGA Professional and Past President of PGA of America Brian Whitcomb.

Many members of our armed forces enlisted at a young age; others are graduates of the various military academies, colleges, and ROTC programs. Each enrolled for a different reason. They serve so that our freedoms are preserved. We must never lose sight of their personal sacrifices. When they return battered and broken, we must assist, as best we can, in their recovery process.

There has always been a great deal of controversy about whether or not we should we go to war. "We may not agree with why we went to this war, previous wars or futures wars," says Vickery, "and I don't care about your opinion on war or if you support war or its cause. But, support the individuals who do serve and come back broken. Support the cause? Maybe or maybe not. Support the person? Absolutely."

These heroes may have shattered bodies, but they don't have shattered spirits. Our sport is extremely adaptable to the disabled person. Golf is like playing on a moving conveyor belt. You can slow down or accelerate. You can get on or off at any time you want because the game moves at your speed. The golf course serves as a bridge, in the needed healing environment, from injury to recovery.

"It is where teaching takes place to help them find happiness in life again and to appreciate what they bring to the table," says Estes.

That healing leads to a refreshed awareness and purpose to their life and, I believe as a golf professional, it is a "fair way" for us to give back. These men and woman who have given their best on the battlefield have inspired me to give them my very best on the golf course. Together we have made outstanding progress in the recovery process. ⚬

The Switch and Release

"You can't just flip the switch the day you get back from war."

There are many men and women who work on Capitol Hill as our senators and representatives. They are Democrats and Republicans, Liberals and Conservatives. They are ensconced in air-conditioned offices wearing tailored business suits, making decisions and passing bills that affect our country.

Conversely, there are the many men and women who serve in the United States Marine Corps. They leave their wives and husbands, mothers and fathers, brothers and sisters, children and grandchildren, friends and jobs. Careers are interrupted and families are forever changed. They are fighting Dust Devils and the enemy, dressed in combat utility uniforms, defending our freedom one M-16 assault rifle at a time.

"The Few, the Proud," as the U.S. Marines are called, are taught to relinquish their individuality for the sake of the team, the squad, the platoon. They go through some of the most rigorous training in the world. Their emphasis is on "Corps Values — honor, courage and commitment."

These proud, committed warriors are ready to "fight anyone, anywhere, within 48 hours," says Marine Corps Reserves Master Sergeant William Gonzalez, who oversees Security Operations at a private country club in Stuart, Florida. He is also a coordinator for Employer Support of Guard and Reserves in Florida.

Marines are taught to be strong, to defend our country, to be prepared for war, and to never let their guard down. Among the training elements encountered prior to defending our nation are marching through water with full packs, rappelling from 60-foot towers and fighting with fixed bayonets, among other challenges. Marines are thoroughly trained prior to deploying to their combat assignments, and once on that field they are at the highest level of intensity.

"We are trained as Marines to be tough," says Gonzalez. "I know many Marines, and men and women in the other branches of the armed forces, who come back from the war and are afraid to ask for assistance. With all the training we get it is almost a sign of weakness if we should have to ask someone else for help — and that could include therapy or taking golf lessons."

There is almost a sense of feeling ashamed to need support. Gonzalez expresses, "I mean, we can't come back and just flip a switch and unwind. It takes time to wind down. We must acclimate out of a state of constant fear, endorphins still running in high gear, and sort out some personal confusion. It's like being in an elevator and dropping 11 floors in a flash. And we are just supposed to deal with things back here when, in fact, we've been out of the loop. It's very hard to do. Hitting golf balls and playing golf is a great release for us. It's a way for us to unwind, let our guard down."

The Marines are known as the "first to fight." If they can survive the Crucible and make it to war and back, then I challenge each Marine to fight for themselves and become involved in a local golf program today.

"Being outside on the golf course is much better than being stuck inside staring at four walls of the rehab center, or at home feeling sorry for myself. I feel like I'm getting a good workout," said a vet I had the opportunity to work with a few years ago while conducting a training session at Camp LeJeune, North Carolina. I have heard this mantra ad infinitum, and each time I do, it makes me proud to be an American and a facilitator of this workout!

Many of the vets I have worked with over the years have found that attending an outdoor golf class can be an extension of their rehabilitation. It is a wonderful place to relieve some stress, and it can evolve into an extremely sociable recreational pastime. I guess you could say golf is the switch to provide a release and enable our returning heroes to finally be "at ease."

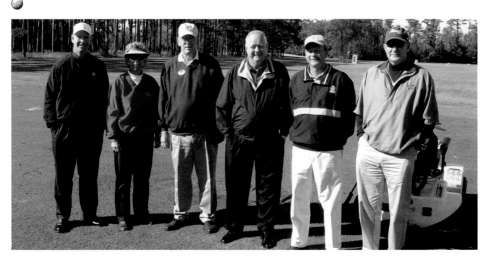

From left to right, PGA Professionals: Jim Ferree, Judy Alvarez, Grant Beck, John Lloyd, Mick Brown and Bruce Oliver, at Camp LeJeune.

Booze 'n Bread

"I guess love letters weren't the only thing being sent in the mail."

It's not every day you have the opportunity to experience the energy of a spirited World War II WAVE, and one whose age matched the day's heat index of 100! On a beastly hot, arid, suffocating June day, I had the pleasure of sharing with Arlene, a most remarkable lady.

Arlene was among a group of active and retired veterans from current and previous combat theaters who had been invited to join us from Walter Reed Army Medical Center. They were attending the Military Appreciation Day Golf Clinic, presented by several local sponsors and the McDonald's LPGA Championship. The event was held at a beautiful private country club in Havre de Grace, Maryland in 2008.

Magnetic, quick-witted Arlene was flanked by four generations of enthusiastic and eager listeners. Our group included LPGA active and retired tour players, staff members from LPGA headquarters, and volunteers from the LPGA Teaching and Club Professionals Division.

Arlene, who had lost her right leg, hunkered down in her four-wheeled red scooter, holding a 7-iron. From this position she proceeded to hold our combined attention as she painted a picture of her many days of service. Arlene was a clerical worker in the United States Navy postal system during days when mail had to be screened. Her duties on her overseas post included administering and sorting through the mail; the safe delivery of the troops' mail between the United States and France was her top priority.

Arlene shared with us that one of the most common items she saw passing through the mail was smuggled booze inside loaves of bread! That was

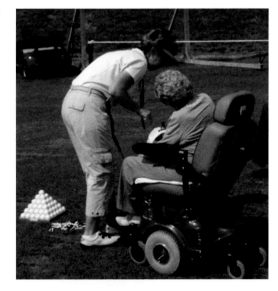

Arlene, a spirited World War II WAVE, receives instruction from Coach Alvarez.

such an odd comment for me to hear. I had never thought about it before, but why would I? I guess love letters were not the only items being sent through the mail in those wartime days!

As I was flying home that night, it occurred to me that the experience of volunteering to give golf lessons continues to provide me with unique and varied experiences. These opportunities are highlighted by the many generations of people brought together because of golf, sharing in healthy outdoor environments, lively laughter, and delightful and engaging stories. This day some received a golf lesson while others had a history lesson.

The Invisible Wound of War
"Golf. Forced Therapy"

You know how you just bond with some people? That's how I felt about Nancy, a calm, poised Petty Office First Class who had served in the Navy for 20 years. We shared a golf cart driving up and down a picturesque country club in New York. Excited to be out in the fresh air, our 18-hole outing was enveloped by calmness. Well, it seemed calm to me; quiet, like virtually any other golf course.

Not for Nancy, who suffers from post-traumatic stress disorder (PTSD). Not that I could tell, however. I wouldn't have even known unless she shared it with me. Let's be honest, unless we can see someone's disability, we don't realize they have one. Nancy is one of the many thousands of vets who come back from war with this invisible disability that manifests itself in anxiety and flashbacks.

I learned of the strength and courage it took for her just to leave the local Medical Center where she was a temporary resident to play golf that day. For most people, the sound of the crack of the driver firing the ball gives a rush of adrenaline in a positive way. For those dealing with PTSD, it's a different ball game. It conjures up the sound of roadside bombings and other horrific experiences.

The day we met, Nancy shared that she had been introduced to golf earlier in the year. She had a few lessons under her belt and we enjoyed the day getting to know one another, comparing stories of my golf career as a female instructor and her life as a woman in the military. I found her a most interesting person.

Nancy shared with me the value of golf to her own rehabilitation and the importance of the game in her recovery.

"Forced therapy," she calls it. "It's a good challenge for me to be out here in this community of golf. I'm safe here, not over there (on the battlefield)." To Nancy, her "invisible wound" is very visible. Through golf, the healing process has begun and each day becomes somewhat easier.

18 Heartfelt and Soulful Memories . . .
A Living Scorecard

As golf instructors, we have the potential to touch a heart and soul in each lesson setting. From that template of a career, I compiled 18 memories of people who stopped in, took a lesson and moved on. Although our encounters were brief and our paths have never crossed again, being exposed to their courage, strength, and confidence touched me and helped shape my teaching in years to come. Our time together helped set the stage for their future as well as my own.

We all have met people who pass briefly through our lives. Some share experiences for a given time. My given times are shared below. I am unsure whether these people know, years later, how much they have touched me as a human being and as an instructor/trainer. These memories remind me that what is between the ears has more weight in strength than muscle, and their inner strength and vision outweigh physical strength every time.

◆ *HOLE No. 1 Somalia's Tears*

Her tears were uncontrollable. I was so moved as I watched this tall, thin teenager see her own golf swing on the split screen next to one of the most famous golfers in the world. People think it's cool to see what their swing looks like next to this tiger of a player, but this experience was somewhat different. She was watching her golf swing for the first time; this was her first exposure to the game of golf. It's amazing what a video camera can do for an individual. It was literally the highlight of her life.

This was one shocker of a lesson for me. A local woman, who was part of a national organization to rescue battered woman from violence in Africa, asked me if I would consider giving a lesson to a girl in her late teens who had lost part of her left arm. I immediately agreed. She continued to confide in me why this lesson was so important to the young lady. The girl had come from Somalia, where she had been beaten, raped and tortured. Her left arm was cut off with a machete just above the elbow. Her right forearm had a huge gash from an unsuccessful attempt to cut it off as well.

I wish you could have seen her light up when the balls she hit went sailing into the air. It was an incredible experience to witness her jumping up and down. It is really amazing to see golf through the eyes of a beginner and to see what golf, in turn, can provide to someone. Her deep raw laughter filled the air. There were quite a few tears shared this day — mostly mine! Our survivor exhibited peace and joy. I know. I saw it on her face and experienced it in a good-bye hug!

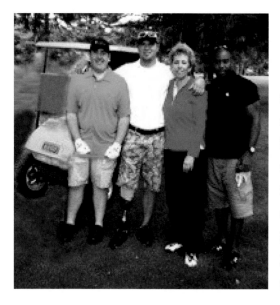

◆ *HOLE No. 2 The Best Foursome to Chase the Ball*

Fun. That's what we had; fun on the golf course. We laughed, cut up and told jokes. We came from different backgrounds and arrived with different experiences. Yet, we were all sharing in the same experience when it came to chasing the ball and trying to get the best score for our team. It was amazing how David, Tim, and Calvin shone at the appropriate time to sink a putt, drive the ball in the fairway, or get it up and down. The chemistry we had wasn't something you buy in a store. Sometimes golf brings strangers together for a few hours of fun, and leaves an indelible mark.

◆ *HOLE No. 3 Career Twist in a Second*

I spent a few hours one day working with George. He was a young man who lost nearly all of the vision in his right eye when an auto antenna pierced his eye socket and exited through his head as he dove for a football while playing street ball in Brooklyn.

George had been a talented, prominent and upcoming tennis player at an early age, though his hopes of raising the U.S. Tennis Open trophy above his head at Flushing Meadows had ended and he'd traded in his dream for a successful career in law. I met George only once; however, I recall how determined he was to hit the ball better in spite of his vision and balance issues. After working on a few swing adjustments and having a few discussions on ball placement positions, George has spent many enjoyable days chasing the dimpled ball with his buddies.

◆ *HOLE No. 4 Heart and Soul of Family Bonding*

When I first met Kevin he was your typical thirteen-year-old, cute, engaging, talking about sports and laughing a lot. The difference was that Kevin had spina bifida. Sitting in a wheelchair, never having swung a golf club before, he worked with me over the hot summer.

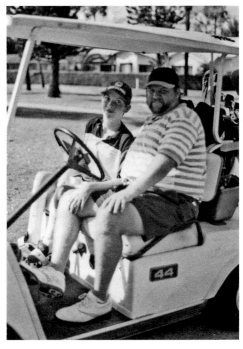

Getting Kevin to make contact with the ball was a good start; hitting the ball 10 to 15 yards was even more outstanding. Kevin also learned how to chip and putt. After numerous operations over the next two years, Kevin was able to drive up to his golf lessons in his own single-rider cart. He was now swinging with two arms and advanced to hitting the ball 50 to 60 yards. He accomplished this with a specially designed 5-wood flattened to 13 degrees, and a special golf glove to help him keep his hands on the club. Kevin's lighthearted expression and roaring laughter showed me that there was much more to golf than just hitting the ball. Kevin showed so much promise that he and his dad, Michael, registered to play as partners in my fourth annual able-bodied/disabled-bodied golf tournament.

Torn between chasing the ball for a few hours together with his son or staying home and watching their favorite football teams play, dad decided to bring a portable TV so they could do both. It was nice watching father and son share something special. This was a day that proved to be the heart and soul of family bonding!

◆ *HOLE No. 5 Hands Down the Best Swing*

Bobbette, a successful doctor, became a partial paraplegic following a near-fatal automobile accident in the late 1980s. Using golf as a rehabilitative tool helped get her life back on track. Now she tackles the game with the most odd, but very effective, finish position I have ever seen. Wearing a brace on a horribly bowed and hyperexteneded left knee, Bobbette walks

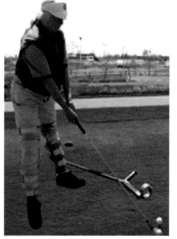

up to the ball with one forearm crutch and a golf club. In preparation to hit the ball, she drops her crutch and carefully achieves her balance. Immediately after striking the ball, her swing is interrupted by collapsing at her hip joints and ends with her hands — still clutching the club in her left hand — flat on the ground, maintaining her knees in a rigid "locked" position to prevent her from buckling and falling.

This display of sheer determination makes me realize that there are endless ways to swing a club, and reminds me to always think outside the box.

(Picture courtesy of Bobbette Ranney)

◆ *HOLE No. 6 Opportunities! Choices! Challenges!*

Opportunities, choices and challenges are without fail always in front of us! Rick, a well-built sergeant, picked up a flyer describing a free golf clinic being offered to wounded warriors of the Brooke Army Medical Center at the Randolph Oaks Golf Course in San Antonio, Texas. The program was run by Disabled Sports USA as part of its Wounded Warrior Disabled Sports Project. PGA Professionals were going to be on hand to offer free golf lessons. Rick made a choice to get away from the stuffy barracks and soak up some fresh air. The biggest challenge was learning how to swing a club with one arm, since he had lost his left arm in the Iraq War. Instead of sliding his lower body from side to side causing the ball to go to the right, we asked him to do two things: keep his lower body still, creating a stable foundation to turn his body on, and add a stronger grip position to help square up the club face.

On this breezy weekday, Rick achieved a sense of accomplishment, released some self-doubt and witnessed how golf can be both a good workout and a stress reliever away from his military quarters.

◆ *HOLE No. 7 Music of Arthritic Golf*

Over the years, I have offered golf classes and taught many private lessons to golfers suffering from arthritis. Since exercise is recommended for people with arthritis, why not play golf? Walking on a golf course is great for your balance, especially with all the hills and undulations. If you are driving a golf cart and feel fatigued, you sit out a hole. No one says you have to play every hole.

To help with absorbing the shock of striking the ball, golfers with arthritis use specially designed padded gloves on both hands, and clubs with fatter grips and graphite shafts. A lower compression golf ball, teed up for all shots as well as for practicing on the driving range, will do wonders for your game. Wear comfortable walking shoes. These simple suggestions will enhance your range of motion and health conditions for your next round of golf.

Donna, one of my students who has undergone multiple bouts of arthritis, says, "It's the sound of nature and hearing the ball hit the bottom of the cup that is the music of golf."

◆ *HOLE No. 8 Introduce a Wide-Topped Tee*

Golf provides a welcome environment for people of all sizes and shapes. A friendly obese man who was addicted to the game of golf came to see me for a lesson. His real issue was not hitting the golf ball; it was the struggle of bending over and trying to balance the ball on a tee. I introduced him to a wide-topped tee and the rest is history.

◆ *HOLE No. 9 Multiple Sclerosis*

Cindy had multiple sclerosis; she knew that regular aerobic exercise increased her fitness and strength and minimized her frustration, anger and fatigue. Cindy desperately wanted to play in a golf outing, yet she tired easily. She was perfect for a scramble format, which provided a safe environment that met all of her needs as well as her limitations. Swinging away, Cindy wore her specially-designed vest, her pockets loaded up with ice packs keeping her cool and energized throughout the day. Her scramble was a success in so many ways!

◆ *HOLE No. 10 Cerebral Palsy*

What I remember most about wiry, lean Marty was that he needed help tying his shoe laces and pulling money out of his wallet to buy a drink at the bar. Compounding the matter, his brain was pumping slurred and spitted words out of his mouth faster than he could react. But when it came to teeing up the ball and striping it down the middle of the fairway, he demonstrated precision. His knock-kneed set up with a text book grip provided him a smooth swing.

Cerebral palsy may have limited Marty in some ways, but when it came to playing golf, he showed ability and the talent to play with the best.

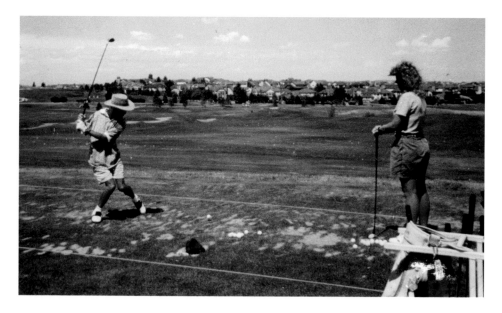

◆ *HOLE No. 11 Sam*

Sam was an independent twelve-year-old when he pitched the winning game to guide his undefeated team to the Little League World Series Championship. As a gift, his parents sent

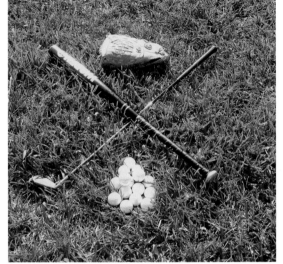

Sam to visit his grandparents' farm for the weekend, a place Sam loved. As he got lost in the fun of the day and was not particularly attentive, Sam's arm became jammed in a tractor.

He woke up in the hospital with half of his pitching arm missing. Years later Sam learned to play one-armed golf, building a swing around his throwing motion. Sam mastered the game of golf and has been playing ever since. He shared with me that although he looks different and misses playing baseball, and even struggles with the loss of his identity, golf taught him that he could still take the curve balls life threw at him as a whole person.

◆ *HOLE No. 12 Dr. M, the Seated One-Armed Swinger*

Dr. M was feeling nauseated and clammy one day, and within 24 hours was paralyzed from the waist down due to an infection in his spine. An avid golfer before his disability, he was in search of a modified golf swing. Using a single rider cart with a thick brown leather strap secured around his abdomen, Dr. M's toes dangled, just touching the ground for some support. From this position he was able to make a full swing with just his right arm, while holding onto the steering handle with his left hand. I personally have seen this man hit the ball 180 yards down the fairway. Good upper body strength and having had the ability to play golf prior to his injury helped. Staying in shape matters!

◆ *HOLE No. 13 Outdoor Parkinson's Therapy*

What a great idea . . . outdoor physical therapy sessions. Once a week, Mark and his wife, a physical therapist, met me under the beige canopy of the narrow driving range. We worked on hitting golf balls, first from his shinny four-wheeled scooter then graduating to a single-rider golf car.

At this point in Mark's life, time spent outside together was more about exercising and "being able to swing without falling over" than completing nine or eighteen holes. In addition to golf maintaining his deteriorating coordination and keeping his muscles active, it was also about getting him out of his house and away from the isolation and feelings of depression. Attempting to hit balls through the tremors and rigidity of Parkinson's was a feat in itself, but I admired Mark's conviction and passion for the game. Not bad for a man who went from shooting 89 for a quarter of a century to appreciating the fact he could still swing a club and get out in the fresh air.

◆ *HOLE No. 14 Green and Bear It*

Anne, one of my golf students, was in the midst of a separation. Sad as she was, the golf course was her refuge and seemed to be the only place where she found solitude. During an on-course playing lesson one day, our time together, brought her game to a new level. As we wrapped it up she said, "Judy, this was the best. With everything that is going on in my life right now, this place is such solitude. It's the only place I can relax and forget about my situation. Thank you! Thank you! Thank you!" She cried as tears streamed down her cheeks.

Where else would one want to "green and bear it" but outside on a beautiful golf course? For all those who have been widowed or are going through a difficult separation or divorce, come visit soon.

◆ *HOLE No. 15 John and Doris Hit Pay Dirt*

John contracted spinal meningitis in the early nineties, which left him a "modified paraplegic." While playing wheelchair tennis one day in the Daytona Beach area, a friend of his told him that "a woman golf pro from down south helped handicap persons with their golf games." John's friend could not remember my name.

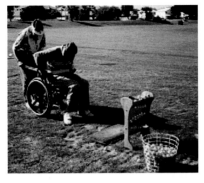

John searched high and low and eventually contacted both The PGA of America and LPGA headquarters. They provided him with my contact information.

John and his wife drove three hours south for a few days of golf lessons. The first thing I wanted to see was how the couple interacted with each other setting up to hit golf balls. I marveled at how Doris secured her husband into his wheelchair. Her use of a luggage strap was incredibly effective! To this day I still recommend using a luggage strap to safely hold someone in a wheelchair.

John sent me a follow-up letter which read in part: "I hit pay dirt when I met you. With a lot of practice and the new clubs that you adjusted for me, my handicap and my scooter for mobility will someday bring me out to the course again. Thank you."

◆ HOLE No. 16 The Vet in Red

The United States Retired Congressman's golf tournament, hosted by the USA Former Members of Congress and benefitting The PGA Military Golf Program and Disabled Sports USA's Wounded Warrior Disabled Sports Project, was held at a private country club in Arlington, Virginia.

One of the players was a stocky, broad-chested bilateral amputee who had lost his legs four months earlier. Wearing a bright red shirt and sporting a flattering square haircut, he joined my foursome for his first round of golf since losing his legs. He was justifiably nervous. The last time he had swung a club he was wearing golf shoes and standing on his own two legs, not strapped into the hydraulic seat of a single-rider golf cart, getting ready to play golf over some strange and intimidating hills for a few hours.

What a joy it was to help this proud soldier and the others that day on the range. The vet in red may have lost his legs, but not his sharp mind or his incredible courage. He accepted the challenge of playing golf with dignity.

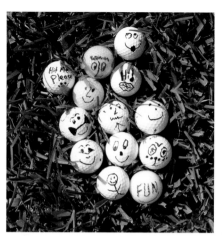

◆ *HOLE No. 17 Funny Faces*

Ten-year-old Julie's attitude was in full swing! This young Special Olympics athlete-to-be was in my care with extreme reluctance. I could just tell she wanted to be anywhere but on the driving range. Yet, her dad was determined to give her a golf lesson, so I tried to make it as much fun as possible for her. It was a losing battle at first, until I found out she had a love for dolls. So... I started drawing smiley faces, funny faces and pictures of dolls on the golf balls. As the pile of pictured golf balls grew for her to choose which one she wanted to hit, so did her smile. In Julie's case, it is the little things in life that go a long way.

◆ *HOLE No. 18 "Ed-ucation"*

I will never forget my experience teaching Ed. I met him when I taught my first eight-week adult educational golf class through the Broward County School System in the winter. He was a talented golfer/athlete with a smooth swing and a great sense of humor. No matter what I tried, I could never get Ed to straighten out his drive, which always catered to the right side of the world.

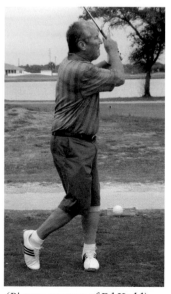

I tried everything I could think of to get him to finish on his front leg, but he just never got his weight all the way over.

One day as spring approached, Ed came to class in a bright yellow baseball cap and checkered shorts. I about fell over. His prosthetic was an "Ed-ucation" for me! I asked him why he had never told me about his leg even though I had asked about any health issues.

He said matter-of-factly, "I didn't think it mattered. I lost it in a motorcycle accident years ago." We talked and we laughed. I guess there are some things golfers prefer to keep private.

(Picture courtesy of Ed Krehl)

Trading In

Many of the stories you have just read are about heroic military men and women who share a common thread. While golf has become an instrumental aspect of their physical rehabilitation and recovery, perhaps golf serves as a greater purpose. The game, in its many adaptations, has given these courageous individuals the opportunity to experience the purity of fresh air and to be the best they can be.

At one point in their lives, each of these people made the choice to trade in the life they knew so that we might all experience a secure and better life. The game of golf has leveled the turf and allowed them to trade in the stress of their disabilities for a beautiful, uplifting and fulfilling experience on the golf course.

Trading In . . .

Combat Boots for Golf Shoes

Guns for Golf Clubs

Campaign Hats for Golf Caps

Fatigues for Golf Shorts and Shirts

Scopes for GPS

Chopper Noise for Chirping Birds

RPG's/IED's for Ball Colliding with Club

Bunkers in the Field for Greenside Bunkers

Camouflage Tents and Mesh Halls for
  Clubhouse

Wheelchairs for Single Rider Carts

Mess Hall for 19th Hole

Battlefields of Stress for Fairways of Lazy
  Afternoon Fun

Isolation from World to Sharing with
  Family and Friends

Pistol Range for Golf Driving Range

Tankers and Humvees for Golf Carts

Chasing the Enemy for Chasing a Golf Ball

VA Hospital for Golf Course

Confidence Obstacle Course for Golf
  Course

Crutches and Canes for Golf Clubs

Fear of the Unknown for Fear of the Known

Hell for Heaven or "Paradise"

Barrage of Mortars for Barrage of Golf Balls

Combat Stress for Beverage Carts

500 Clicks for 500 Yards

Shrapnel for Wooden Tees

Dust Devils of Iraq for Green Grass

Deadly Hazards for Golf Hazards

Nightmares for Day Dreams

Addiction to Drugs for Addiction to Life
  and Golf

Sinking Hearts for Sinking Putts

Depression for Happiness

Hospital Hallways for Fairways

Drill Instructor for Golf Instructor

Crucible- 54 Hour Challenge for 18 Holes -
  4 Hours

Sharing Quarters for Sharing Scores

Swamp March for March to the Green

Sergeants and Generals for Caddies and
  Marshalls

Circling Back for the Back Nine

Enemy Flag for Golf Flagstick

The 19th Hole

You have met many people within the margins of this book, each illustrating the progress made within the accessible golfing community. As you will recall, when I started teaching golf to the disabled 20 years ago, there was an accessible golf "black hole" for both the instructor and the consumer.

We have come a long way over the years; however, we still have many long fairways ahead of us. I will not feel at ease until there is as rich a directory of accessible golf programs available to the consumer as there are women's and juniors' programs. We need to offer specialized training and advanced "accessible golf" certification to PGA and LPGA Professionals. This training could be modeled after instructor seminars for adaptive skiing. We should strive for better communication between the health care industry and the golfing community.

It is my hope that *Broken Tees and Mended Hearts* helps swing open a new door to provide a nationwide accessible golf "blanket" to honor our wounded warriors and injured spirits, and possibly involve you as well.

Compared to previous combat theaters, many more thousands of military men and women are staying alive and surviving traumatic events, due to exponential advancements in modern technology. We have a generation of amputees returning home to our communities from the wars in Iraq and Afghanistan. From new and improved body armor, like Kevlar vests and helmets, to better-equipped Humvees featuring armored doors with bullet-resistant glass, side and rear armor plates, and ballistic windshields, our military heroes are being rescued from the battlefield at a faster rate. Their survival also is the result of the benefits of military helicopters outfitted with essential medical equipment and care. They are then transported to a nearby hospital with life-sustaining equipment, where nurses and doctors can perform immediate surgery.

As few as 10 days from battlefield injury, the wounded can be stateside, at one of many medical centers, including Walter Reed Army Medical Center, where they begin their rehab. Within weeks, they can be fitted for some of the most advanced prosthetics. We also have an estimated 300,000[1] soldiers returning home from battle having suffered the invisible wound of war — post-traumatic stress disorder (PTSD).

Furthermore, as we mark the 20th anniversary of the Americans with Disability Act, our country has approximately 54 million Americans who are disabled[2]. Add to the mix roughly 76 million Baby Boomers who will begin turning 65 in 2011 and entering retirement[3]. Now, more than ever in our history, it is time to provide accessible golf programs for these patriots and our aging population.

The Department of Justice is reviewing whether to mandate new guidelines governing golf course operators to make available single-rider golf carts at their facilities.

Presently, we have Patriot Golf Day and events conducted year round by Tee It Up For the Troops and the National Amputee Golf Association. Other organizations across the country are embracing golf courses as a therapeutic backbone, underscoring the fact that healing progresses faster in a welcoming outdoor environment. Unlike the battlefield, our playing field is a salvation to those who have endured medical and life-altering hardships. It provides the opportunity for veterans to be free of walls, hallways, and medical settings by stepping on to a practice range.

If you have come this far along the journey, you are now at a most popular port of call for any golfer — the 19th hole. Pull up a stool, let me buy you your favorite clubhouse beverage, and we can reminisce about what you have gathered from these inspirational stories.

Golf welcomes everyone regardless of age, gender, economic status, ability or disability, disease, or injury, and features its own rehabilitative "aura" for anyone recovering from injury or living with a disability.

Golf has enhanced the quality of these individuals' lives on and off the golf course. We also learned that the golf arena provides a safe haven for people to deal with emotional scars, such as PTSD, going through a divorce or losing a spouse.

We have witnessed how the game of golf can have a positive influence on someone's life regardless of disability/injury. We have teed it up with those who live with strokes, spinal cord injuries, arthritis, back injuries, multiple sclerosis, Parkinson's disease, spina bifida, cerebral

[1] Martin, D, 2010. PTSD Treatment access to get easier for veterans.
http://www.cbsnews.com/stories/2010/07/12/eveningnews/main6671863.shtml
[2] 2010 Facts for Features, Newsroom, U.S. Census Bureau
www.census.gov/newsroom
[3] Hagga, J, Population Reference Bureau 2002. Just How Many Baby Boomers Are There?
http://www.prb.org/Articles/2002/JustHowManyBabyBoomersAreThere.aspx

palsy, Down syndrome, muscular dystrophy, myasthenia gravis, cancer, asthma, traumatic brain injury, and more.

Like a needle and thread, we can use the game of golf to bind people with disabilities and injuries together with PGA/LPGA instructors and health care providers.

Golf promotes the platform to individuality, independence, self-esteem, and self-confidence. That avenue to improvement may be rolling balls on the putting green, spending hours on the practice range, chasing the ball on the course or just sharing a bite to eat with a friend overlooking some tranquil scenery from the clubhouse.

I am sure you will remember how learning to swing from a seated position helped renew Herb and Sue's life on the golf course after his paralysis, and how Dan discovered that if he could hit golf balls off one leg, he most probably could tackle anything life threw at him. Cancer may have struck Stan, but it also afforded him quality time with his children on the golf course. Gail, who survived a plane crash, is still playing golf in all corners of the country with her friends and family. Her generosity allows organizations to use her golf course to raise funds for charitable causes. It's hard to forget John, who awoke from a coma after electrocution had ravaged his body, and relied on golf to guide him through 109 surgeries. We also met Vicki, who showed us that the hardest door to walk out of is your own front door.

For all those military men and women who chose to proudly don a uniform and stand in harm's way to protect our country's principles and liberties of freedom, I salute you!

For all those who showed me the intangible qualities the game of golf offers by demonstrating incredible courage, strength, perseverance, and will, you have my utmost respect and admiration, and I thank you!

Share these titanic positives with someone you love today and make a difference in his or her life, one swing at a time. There are countless people across the country who can benefit from the game of golf as a rehabilitative tool and recreational outlet.

Whether you're an enthusiastic golfer, a motivated instructor, an avid reader or someone who wants to make a difference in the life of someone else, I hope you're asking, "How can I help? What can I do? How do I find an accessible golf program?" You can begin by reviewing the "Accessible Golf Ambassador Call to Action Plan."

Without doubt, have conviction and fortitude; reach out and lend a hand. Imagine the impact you will have on those you love. If you act on just one suggestion from the Ambassador list on the next page you will see a remarkable difference.

As we travel the fairways of our lives, may our paths converge, our swings improve and our mission remain clear — we will bring healing to all through GOLF, the game we love.

Your caddie,

Judy Alvarez, PGA/LPGA

Accessible Golf Ambassador Call to Action Plan

❑ Donate to a charitable organization listed in the Resource Guide.

❑ Volunteer your time to a local accessible golf program or charity, Wounded Warrior Project or Disabled Sports USA.

❑ If you are a PGA/LPGA golf professional, start an accessible golf program at your facility.

❑ If you are a course operator, host or start your own inclusion golf event.

❑ Register to be an official Patriot Golf Day host facility (Labor Day Weekend) or play golf this weekend and donate a minimum of $1.

❑ Philanthropically support one of the organizations listed in the Resource Guide.

❑ Host a fundraising event at your local golf course.

❑ Play in or host an event for Tee It Up For the Troops.

❑ Invite members of the Armed Forces to your club for a day.

❑ Invite patients from local rehab centers to your club for a golf clinic.

❑ Provide this book as a tournament gift or handout to patients at one of 137 VA hospitals nationwide, or in rehab centers.

❑ Encourage your staff to read these motivational stories whether you are a Fortune 500 company, non-profit organization, small business or Chamber of Commerce.

❑ Team with golf and military and non-military healthcare professionals on projects for your golf students/patients.

❑ If you have stopped playing golf, get back into the game today.

❑ If you have been thinking about playing the game of golf, contact your local PGA/LPGA Professional today.

❑ If you have a loved one or friend sitting home depressed, lonely or disabled, invite them to a golf course today, even if it is just for lunch!

❑ Invite National Amputee Golf Association's First Swing Golf Clinics to your facility.

❑ If you have a disability or injury, reach out to any of the organizations listed in the Resource Guide.

❑ PGA/LPGA Professionals should pause and review other models of successful accessible sports programs (skiing, wheelchair tennis, basketball).

Resource Guide *

Additional Life Links and Intervention

* This guide is not exhaustive and does not formally recommend or endorse the equipment and organization(s) listed. Individuals should investigate and determine on their own which equipment and organization(s) best fits their needs.

Accessible Golf Programs Listed by State

California (Northern)
American Heart/American Stroke Association
www.savingstrokes.com

Colorado
www.golf4fun.org/

Florida
Adaptive Golf Academy
www.adaptivegolfacademy.com

Illinois
Marionjoy Rehabilitation Hospital Therapeutic Golf Program
www.marianjoy.org/

Iowa
Golf For Injured Veterans Everywhere G.I.V.E.
www.giveforveterans.com

Kansas
Buddie's Veterans Accessible Golf
www.buddiesbuddies.org

Maryland
Salute Military Golf Association
www.smga.org

Kernan Hospital Golf Clinics
www.hernan.org/rehabilitation/golf

Michigan
Flint Adaptive Golf at McLaren Regional Rehabilitation Center
www.mclarenregional.org/body

Minnesota
Sister Kenny Golf Program
www.allina.com

Montana
Eagle Mount Billings Accessible Golf Program
www.eaglemount.us/

Nevada
Las Vegas Adaptive Recreation Division
www.lasvegasnevada.gov

New York
Helen Hayes Hospital Golf Ability Program
www.helenhayeshospital.org/special_services/golfability.htm

Ohio
Edwin Shaw Rehabilitation Institute Challenge Golf
www.akrongeneral.org

Fore Hope www.forehope.org/

Golf Without Handicap (Cleveland Sight Center)
www.clevelandsightcenter.org

Pennsylvania
Eastern Amputee Golf Association
http://www.eaga.org/

Accessible Golf Programs Nationwide

Disabled Sports USA
104 chapters in 37 states
www.dsusa.org

G.A.I.N. (Golf: Accessible and Inclusive Networks)
www.accessgolf.org/gain

Golf courses owned by the Government
(municipal, city, county, state, military
bases)
Search by: accessible golf, adaptive golf,
recreation department, special populations

National Amputee Golf Association First
Swing Learn to Golf Clinics
www.nagagolf.org

Military and non military golf programs
Play Golf America (PGA)
www.playgolfamerica.com

To locate a PGA/LPGA golf instructor in
your area contact:
LPGA
www.lpga.com

Mobility Golf
www.mobilitygolf.com

PGA of America
www.pgaofamerica.com

USGA
www.usga.org

To locate accessible golf courses and
tournaments in your area:
Mobility Golf
www.mobilitygolf.com

National Alliance for Accessible Golf
www.accessgolf.org

National Amputee Golf Association
www.naga.org

Tee It Up For The Troops
www.teeitupforthetroops.com

Golf and Related Associations
American Disabled Golfers Association
www.americandisabledgolfersassociation.
com

Club Managers Association of America
www.cmaa.org

Disabled American Veterans
www.dav.org

Disabled Sports USA
www.dsusa.org

Folds of Honor Foundation
www.foldsofhonor.org

Golf Course Superintendents Association of
America
www.gcsaa.org

Ladies Professional Golf Association
www.lpga.com

Limbs For Life Foundation
www.limbsforlife.org

National Alliance for Accessible Golf
www.resourcecenter.usga.org

National Golf Course Owners Association
www.ngcoa.org

National Golf Foundation
www.ngf.org

Paralympics
www.usparalympics.org

Paralyzed Veterans of America
www.pva.org

PGA of America
www.pgafoundation.org
www.playgolfamerica.com

Special Olympics
www.specialolympics.org

The Dennis Walters Show
www.denniswaltershow.com

The Sentinels of Freedom
www.sentinelsoffreedom.org

United States Blind Golf Association
www.usblindgolf.com

United States Deaf Golf Association
www.usdeafgolf.org/

United States Golf Association Resource
Center for Individuals with Disabilities
www.resourcecenter.usga.org

Wounded Warrior Project
www.woundedwarriorproject.org

Amputee Associations
Amputee Coalition of America
www.amputee-coalition.org

Canadian Amputee Golf Association
www.caga.ca

Eastern Amputee Golf Association
www.eaga.org

Midwestern Amputee Golf Association
www.mwaga.org

National Amputee Golf Association
www.naga.org

North American One-Armed Golf
Association
www.naoaga.com

Southern Amputee Golf Association
www.sagagolf.com

Western Amputee Golf Association
www.wagagolf.com

Recreation Organizations Related to Golf
Adaptive Information Resource Center
www.adaptiveirc.org/sports/golfN.html

American Therapeutic Recreation
Association (ATRA)
www.atra-tr.org

Arthritis Foundation
www.arthritis.org/golf

National Center on Accessibility
www.ncaonline.org

National Center on Physical Activity and
Disability
www.ncpad.org

National Recreation and Parks Association
(NRPA)
www.nrpa.org

United States Association of Blind Athletes
www.usaba.org

Other
Americans with Disabilities Act (ADA)
www.adata.org

Information and Resources for Persons with
Disabilities (Disaboom)
www.disaboom.com

United States Access Board
www.access-board.gov

U.S. Department of Justice
www.ada.gov/regs2010/ADAregs2010.htm

U.S. Department of Veterans Affairs
www.va.gov

Publications
Accessible Golf Fore All (LPGA Publication)

Amputee Golfer Magazine
www.nagagolf.org

Challenge Golf (PGA Publication)
www.pga.com

Instructional Tips for Golfers with Disabilities
by Judy Alvarez
www.indiana.edu/~nca/ncpad/golftips.
shtml

Paraplegia News: Sports 'n Spokes
www.pvamagazines.com/pnnews

USGA Modified Rules of Golf (Golfers with
Disabilities)
www.usga.org/rules/disabilities

Adaptive Golf Equipment Resources

Adaptive Gloves, Grip Aids, Prosthetic Arm Grip Devices

Amputee Golf Grip (prosthetic arm attachment)
www.oandp.com/trs

BOINIC Gloves (padded glove for arthritic conditions)
www.bionicgloves.com

Formed Golf Training Grip (memory aid for correct golf grip)
www.golfaroundtheworld.com

Grip Mate (gripping device for hands with no fingers)
www.gripmate.com

Grip Wrap (gripping strap for securing one or both hands to club)
www.golfaroundtheworld.com

Hanger Prosthetics & Orthotics
www.hanger.com

Power Glove (golf glove with loop to secure golf grip to glove)
www.powerglove.com

Sport Aid Arm Device (prosthetic arm attachment, golf arm gripping device)
www.nextstepoandp.com

Therapeutic Recreation Services, Inc. (amputee golf grips)
www.oandp.com/products/trs/

Single Rider Golf Carts

Eagle Products
www.eagleproducts.com

Electric Mobilty
www.electricmobility.com

Fairway Golf Car
www.fairwaygolfcarts.com

Golf Express
www.golfexpress.com

HiRider
www.falconrehab.net/products

Mobility Golf
www.mobilitygolf.com

Pride Mobility
www.pridemobility.com

Solorider
www.solorider.com

Stand Up and Play
www.standupandplay.org

Static Chair (for someone that can stand but with poor balance such as a stroke)
www.usagpi.com

Adaptive Golf Clubs

Golf Ball Grabber (device for picking up golf ball)
www.thatsclever.com

Matzie Golf Company
www.matzie.com

Pat Ryan Golf (adaptive golf clubs)
www.patryangolf.com

The Professional Clubmakers Society (adaptive golf clubs for seated golfer)
www.proclubmakers.org

Toteinbonezgolf (adaptive golf clubs for seated golfer)
www.toteinbonezgolf.com

UPRIGHT Golf (accessible golf clubs for seated golfer)
www.uprightgolf.com

Other
Access to Recreation
www.accesstr.com

Achievable Concepts
www.achievableconcepts.com

EZT Golf Ball Feeder (self teeing devices for total independence)
www.usagpi.com

Golf Country (adaptive golf supplies)
www.golf-country.com

UPRIGHT Golf (accessible devices: golf ball grabber, teeing devices, putter suction cups, etc.)
www.uprightgolf.com

Grants and Funding
Access to Recreation
www.accesstr.com

Florida Junior Golf Council
www.fjgc.org

National Alliance for Accessible Golf
www.accessgolf.org

PGA of America
www.pgafoundation.com

Juniors
Creative Solutions for Amputees (upper extremity girls and woman)
www.cs4a.org

Junior Golf Information
www.childrensgolf.org

Kids in Disability Sports, Inc.
www.kidsindisabiltysports.com

Middle Atlantic Blind Golfers Association (junior golf program)
www.mabga.org

S.N.A.G. (fun teaching aids for all ages)
www.snaggolf.com

The First Tee
www.thefirsttee.org

U.S. Kids Golf (equipment for juniors)
www.uskidsgolf.com

Acknowledgements and Thanks

This book did not come to life on its own. I would have been a ship lost at sea had I not received the support on some capacity from everyone listed below.

My "Foursome":

Player No. 1: God

My constant companion who is always there to support me in moments of weakness, frustration, excitement and joy. He pulled me through like He always does. Thank you.

Player No. 2: Bob Denney, Editor

Bob, I know we had spoken about collaborating on a book project for quite some time, but the timing on my part to undertake a project of this magnitude never seemed right. Thank you for taking me aside at the PGA Merchandise Show in Orlando, and igniting the switch. That night, I wrote my first story, A Moment of Impact. Teeing it up with you over the last two years has been a wonderful experience. Thank you for all your support, effort and vision. You have always come through for me.

Player No. 3: Suzanne Boehmcke, "Junior" Editor

Suzanne, if it were not for you I would still be writing this book. You were truly one of the driving forces behind the completion of this project. Thank you for organizing my thoughts and ideas. I couldn't have done this without you. I will always remember my trip to Long Island. You will always have a special place in my heart. I owe you so much. Thank you very, very much.

Player No. 4: Judy Ellis, Graphic Designer

Judy, I am not sure you knew what you were getting into when you offered to help me with this project, but I am extremely grateful. I appreciate your vision and tenacity in helping make this book come alive. Thank you.

Special Thank You

A noteworthy thank you to Greg Jones for having the vision to form the now defunct Association of Disabled American Golfers. You were ahead of your time. Had it not been for you, I might still be searching for ways to teach golf to the disabled. May you rest in peace. I hope you knew that what you started was only the beginning. You are missed.

A special thank you to Mariner Sands Country Club members and staff:, PGA Director of Golf, Tim McKenna, PGA Head Golf Professional, Jim Chorniewy, Pat Ross, Karen Das and PGA Professional Sean Pender. Thank you for putting up with me for months on end. To so many wonderful and supporting members who provided encouragement. Thank you to everyone who listened to my many "play-by-play" updates on the status of the book. I appreciate each and every one of you. Thank you!

Thank you to Gene Gillis for your time and effort in creating, editing and maintaining my website.

I would be remiss if I did not mention and thank the following people for helping me in some capacity over the years, whether it was helping me comb the country to find people I lost contact with as far back as 20 years ago, making a telephone call or sending an email on my behalf. To others, thank you for influencing my teaching career and supporting me over the years:

Sonny Ackerman, Ronald Alvarez, Ph.D., Elaine Alvarez, Dan Alvarez, Jennifer Atkisson-Lovett, LPGA Professional Marsha Bailey, Executive Director Disabled Sports USA Kirk Bauer, Past National President of LPGA and LPGA Professional Patti Benson, Jim Brown, Betsy Clark, Ph. D., Julie Costa (my Jr. Jr. editor), Caylin Costa, Kevin Costa, Nancy Costa, Jeff Ellis, James Fenton, Susan Frasca, LPGA Professional and LPGA T&CP Executive Director Nancy Henderson, Cindy Jones, Steve Jubb, LPGA Master/Life Professional Pat Lang, Tim Lang, LPGA Professional and World Golf Hall of Fame Member Carol Mann, PGA Master Professional Rick Martino, Jerry May, Betty Michalewicz, LPGA Professional DeDe Owens, Ph. D., Scott Parratto, MD, PGA Master Professional Conrad Rehling, President Access Solutions Group LLC Gary Robb, Josephine Scanlon, Mike and Tappy Scanlon, Jeff Searcy, PGA Professional Craig Shankland, Dick and Roz Steinberg, Dan Shube, Chief Executive Officer of PGA of America Joseph Steranka, Richard Thesing, Henry Thrower, Kim Van Buskirk, HB Warren, LPGA Professional Donna White, Past President of PGA of America and PGA Professional Brian Whitcomb, NAGA Executive Director Bob Wilson, President of The PGA of America and PGA Professional Allen Wronowski.

Thank you to all my golf students and the many people who volunteered for the Brighter Fairways Golf Classic. Thank you to the many thousands of military men and woman who have served in our Armed Forces to protect the borders of our country's freedom.

Thank you to the members and staff of The PGA of America and LPGA, Folds of Honor Foundation, Disabled Sports USA, National Amputee Golf Association, Palm Beach County Parks and Recreation Department, Salute Military Golf Association, Tee It Up For The Troops and Walter Reed Army Medical Center.

Index

This Index serves as a means to direct you to stories and resources related to specific conditions, disabilities and disorders. However, as is often the case, many of these overlap. It is my hope that you will take the time to read each individual's story to learn, not only the challenges they overcame, but the courage and strength they found, which can be used to battle any obstacle.

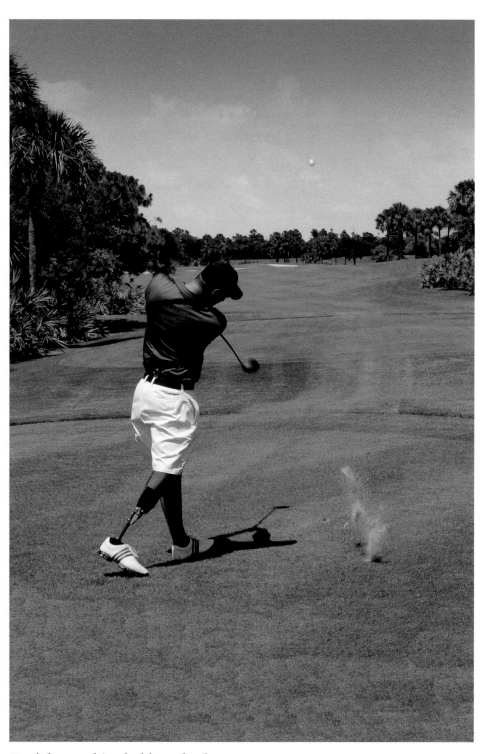

Don't let anything hold you back.
USMC Retired Lance Cpl. Tim Lang (Picture by Jeff Ellis)